AF726076

FENBENDAZOLE & IVERMECTIN PROTOCOLS EXPLAINED FOR SENIORS

WHAT THE RESEARCH REALLY SHOWS ABOUT CANCER CLAIMS, MEDICATION RISKS, AND INFORMED DECISIONS WITH YOUR ONCOLOGY TEAM

ELEANOR WHITMORE

WHITMORE PUBLISHING

CONTENTS

Introduction vii

1. BEFORE YOU TRUST AN ONLINE PROTOCOL 1
Taking the Claim Apart from the Story Around It 1
When Something Looks Like Evidence but Is Not 2
The Evidence Ladder and What Each Rung Can Answer 3
Why Laboratory Plausibility Is Not a Clinical Outcome 6
Why an Anecdote Can Matter Without Proving Anything 7
Approved, Off-Label, Investigational, Veterinary 8
Reading a Trial for What It Actually Measured 9
When More Than One Thing Is Happening at Once 12
Publication Is Not the Finish Line 13
The Claim Check, Expanded 14
What This Chapter Does Not Ask of You 15
Where This Leads 16

2. FENBENDAZOLE: WHAT THE EVIDENCE ACTUALLY SHOWS 17
What This Compound Is 17
Why Researchers Became Interested 18
What the Laboratory and Animal Research Has Shown 19
Why the Gap to Humans Is Especially Wide Here 21
What Human Evidence Exists 22
The Account That Started This 24
What the Published Case Reports Show 25
Why the Protocols Vary 27
The Safety Questions Nobody Has Answered 28
What Would Have to Change 30
Six Questions Worth Asking 33
Where This Leads 34

3. IVERMECTIN AND MEBENDAZOLE: A MORE COMPLICATED PICTURE 35
Why These Two Get Grouped With the First 35
Ivermectin: What It Is and Why the Interest Arose 36
The Concentration Question 37
What Human Trials of Ivermectin Have Found 39
Mebendazole: What It Is and Why the Interest Arose 40
What Human Trials of Mebendazole Have Found 42
The Cohort Study Everyone Is Citing 44
What "Approved and Safe" Does and Does Not Buy You 47
Three Compounds, Side by Side 49

Why Evidence Cannot Be Passed Between Them 49
When They Are Taken Together 51
Three Verdicts, Stated Separately 52
Six Questions Worth Asking 53
Where This Leads 54

4. SAFETY IS NOT A PROPERTY OF A COMPOUND 55
Why "Is It Safe?" Cannot Be Answered 55
What the Previous Chapters Established, and Where It Runs Out 56
Age Is Not the Variable That Matters 57
What Actually Changes 58
The Complete Medication Picture 60
How Interactions Actually Work 61
The Pump That Protects Your Brain 63
Overlapping Effects 64
What Monitoring Can and Cannot Do 65
What "Unstudied" Actually Means 67
Why "Natural" and "Well Tolerated" Mislead Here 67
Eight Questions Worth Asking 72
If You Are Already Taking Something 73
Where This Leads 73

5. TURNING WHAT YOU KNOW INTO A CONVERSATION 75
The Only Place This Can Be Settled 75
Freezing the Claim 76
The Claim Brief 77
What Else to Bring 78
Questions That Produce Answers 78
When the Answer Is "I Don't Know" 80
When It Goes Badly 80
Who Can Help With What 82
Second Opinions 84
Between Appointments 85
Clinical Trials 86
Warning Signs 87
Where This Leaves You 89
Where This Leads 90

6. WHAT TO CARRY WITH YOU 91
Back to the Link 91
What the Evidence Came To 92
What Hope Is For 93
What This Book Did Not Do 94
The Last Thing 95

COPYRIGHT AND MEDICAL DISCLAIMER

Fenbendazole & Ivermectin Protocols Explained for Seniors

What the Research Really Shows About Cancer Claims, Medication Risks, and Informed Decisions With Your Oncology Team

First Edition, 2026

Published by: **Whitmore Publishing**

MEDICAL DISCLAIMER

This book is provided solely for educational and informational purposes. It does not constitute medical advice, diagnosis, treatment, prescription, or an individualized assessment of risks and benefits. Reading this book does not create a clinician–patient relationship.

The discussion of fenbendazole, ivermectin, mebendazole, supplements, repurposed medicines, investigational approaches, off-label uses, online protocols, case reports, or patient experiences is descriptive and analytical only. Inclusion does not constitute endorsement or a recommendation to use any substance for cancer or any other condition.

Do not use this book to start, stop, delay, replace, combine, or change cancer treatment, prescription medication, over-the-counter medication, supplements, or dosages. Never use a product labeled for animals in yourself or another person. Decisions concerning treatment or medication must be made with an appropriately qualified healthcare professional who knows the patient's medical history, current treatments, medications, supplements, allergies, laboratory findings, and individual circumstances.

This is especially important when multiple medications or health conditions are involved. Age alone does not determine risk, and the information in this book cannot predict how any particular person will respond to a medication, supplement, or treatment.

Scientific and medical knowledge changes over time. Although reasonable care has been taken to represent the available evidence accurately as of the publication date, studies may later be corrected, retracted, reinterpreted, or superseded. Regulatory approvals and clinical-trial statuses may also vary by country and change after publication. No guarantee is made that the information is complete, current, or free from error.

Personal stories, case reports, laboratory findings, animal studies, and early clinical research do not establish that a treatment is safe or effective for an individual patient. Outcomes described in any source should not be interpreted as typical, guaranteed, or predictive.

The author and publisher disclaim warranties concerning the use of this information and, to the fullest extent permitted by applicable law, accept no responsibility for injury, loss, or damage

INTRODUCTION

WHY YOU'RE HERE, AND WHAT THIS BOOK WILL HELP YOU DO

Someone sent you a link.

Maybe it was a video with a title in capital letters. Maybe it was a screenshot of a post, forwarded by a cousin who meant well. Maybe you found it yourself, late at night, after the rest of the house had gone quiet and the search box was the only thing still awake. The claim was simple and it was enormous. A cheap, ordinary drug, the kind sold for deworming animals or treating parasites, is quietly curing cancer, and the people who are supposed to be helping you have not mentioned it.

If you are reading this, you did not simply accept that claim. You also did not simply throw it away. You did something harder. You decided to find out what is actually known.

That is the right instinct, and this book is built for it.

You may be the person with the diagnosis. You may be the husband, wife, son, daughter, sister, neighbor, or friend who has taken on the job of reading everything so that someone you love does not have to. Either way, you are probably tired. There may be a stack of appointment notes on the kitchen table, a list of medicines longer than it used to be, and a phone that keeps delivering new videos on the same subject. Under those conditions a simple story is powerfully appealing. It offers something the medical system rarely offers, which is a clear answer, available immediately, with no waiting room.

This book will not hand you that kind of answer, because in this particular subject that kind of answer does not exist. What it offers instead is something more durable. It will teach you how to take a claim of this type apart and find out exactly what is known, what is uncertain, and what has never been studied at all. That skill does not expire when the current viral claim fades. The next one is already being filmed.

WHY THESE STORIES ARE SO CONVINCING

It is worth pausing on why these accounts land as hard as they do, because the reason is not gullibility.

A good protocol story has a shape that human beings are built to find persuasive. There is a named person with a diagnosis and a date. There is a moment when everything looked hopeless. There is a simple intervention, and then there is recovery. The story has a hero, and it usually has a villain in the background. Several of its details are also verifiably true, which is what gives the rest of it credibility. The drugs really are inexpensive. They really have been used safely for decades in their approved settings. Laboratory studies really have found activity against cancer cells, and those papers really are published in real journals with real authors.

What the story leaves out is everything that did not happen. You do not see the people who tried the same thing and died anyway, because they are not making videos. You do not see the conventional treatment that was running at the same time. You do not see how many people took the compound and had no measurable change. What reaches you is the small number of accounts that came out well, which makes an unusual outcome look like a typical one.

None of that means the people sharing these stories are dishonest. Most of them are sincere, and many are frightened. Sincerity is simply not the same thing as evidence, and the two are easy to confuse when you are exhausted and someone is offering hope.

If you are the family member doing the research, this is also where your role is most valuable and most delicate. You can gather sources, keep track of dates, and prepare questions. What you cannot do, and should not try to do, is decide on someone else's behalf. Ask the person how much they want to know and how involved they want you to be, and let their answer govern. The goal is a better-informed decision made by the person whose body it is.

WHY THESE NAMES TRAVEL TOGETHER

Three drug names come up again and again in these conversations: fenbendazole, ivermectin, and mebendazole. Online, they are often discussed as though they were one thing, or as though they were three versions of the same thing.

It is not hard to see why they ended up grouped. All three are antiparasitic medicines. All three are inexpensive. All three have been used for decades, which makes them feel familiar and low-risk. None of them is a new product from a large drug company, which fits a story many people already believe about who benefits from what. And each of them has generated laboratory research suggesting activity against cancer cells, which supplies the grouping with a scientific-sounding foundation.

But the grouping is a fact about the internet, not a fact about pharmacology. It describes how these names travel together in videos and forum posts. It does not describe how the compounds behave in a human body, and it does not mean that evidence about one tells you anything about another.

This is the first idea this book will ask you to hold onto, and it is the one that most often gets lost.

Three Compounds, Three Separate Bodies of Evidence

Here is where the three drugs actually stand in the United States as of this book's research cutoff.

Ivermectin is an approved human medicine. In tablet form it is approved to treat two specific parasitic infections: intestinal strongyloidiasis and onchocerciasis, also called river blindness [SRC-0001]. It is a real prescription drug with a real label, a documented safety record in its approved uses, and known interactions.

Mebendazole is also an approved human medicine. It has been approved in the United States since 1974 for common intestinal worm infections, and it remains available today by prescription for pinworm, whipworm, roundworm, and hookworm [SRC-0002, SRC-0003].

Fenbendazole is different. In the United States it is approved as a veterinary drug. It is a dewormer for cattle, goats, dogs, horses, and other animals, and new veterinary versions of it continue to be approved [SRC-0004]. There is no approved human formulation and no approved human use, which also means there is no regulator-reviewed human labeling for it [SRC-0005].

And here is the point that matters most: none of the three is approved to treat any cancer.

That single sentence does a great deal of work, so it is worth being precise about what it does and does not mean. It does not mean these compounds are worthless, fraudulent, or unworthy of study. It does not mean that scientists who have investigated them were wasting their time. It means only what it says. No regulator has reviewed evidence and concluded that any of these drugs has been shown to treat cancer in people.

Approval is always approval *for something*. A drug approved for a parasitic infection has been evaluated for that infection, at that exposure, in those patients. It has not been evaluated as a cancer treatment. "Approved for humans" and "approved for cancer" are two entirely different statements, and online they are constantly blurred into one.

A related confusion runs in the opposite direction. Some readers conclude that because a compound is used in animals, the whole subject is absurd. That reaction is understandable, and it is also wrong. A veterinary origin says nothing about whether a molecule is scientifically interesting. Plenty of medicines are used in both animals and people, and researchers investigate compounds from all sorts of starting points. Scientific interest is a legitimate thing to have. What a veterinary approval cannot do is establish that a product made for a cow or a dog is suitable for a person with cancer, at a different exposure, over a different length of time. Those are separate questions, and dismissing the first does not answer the second.

There is one more distinction to carry with you from the start, and it may be the most important one in the entire book. Showing that a compound kills cancer cells in a laboratory dish and showing that it helps a patient live longer are not the same finding, and they are not even close. They answer different questions, using different methods, with different things capable of going wrong. A great many compounds kill cancer cells in a dish. Most of them never become treatments, and the reasons are not conspiratorial. Chapter 1 explains exactly where the gap between those two findings opens up.

The same discipline applies between the three compounds. Fenbendazole and mebendazole are chemically related, both belonging to a family called the benzimidazoles, but they are not the same drug and they are not interchangeable. Human research on mebendazole is evidence about mebendazole. Ivermectin is not a benzimidazole at all and belongs to a different chemical class entirely, so evidence about it cannot be carried across to either of the others. When a video answers a question about fenbendazole by citing a trial of mebendazole, something has quietly gone wrong, and later chapters will show you exactly how to spot it.

WHY AGE CHANGES THE QUESTIONS, NOT THE STANDARD OF PROOF

This is a book written with older adults and their families specifically in mind. That deserves an explanation, because the phrase "for seniors" is sometimes used to mean "simplified" or "watered down." That is not what is happening here.

Age changes which questions become important. It does not change how much evidence a claim needs before it can be believed.

Start with what age does not mean. It does not mean frailty. It does not mean confusion, dependence, or an inability to weigh a decision. Plenty of people in their seventies and eighties are managing their own care, reading primary research, and asking their oncologists sharper questions than their doctors expect. Chronological age is not a diagnosis, and the current professional guidance in cancer care reflects exactly that. It recommends that specific factors such as physical function, other medical conditions, nutrition, cognition, and medication use be *assessed* in each individual rather than assumed from a birth date [SRC-0006].

What is more common with age is complexity. Among older adults with advanced cancer starting a new treatment, taking five or more medicines is the norm rather than the exception, and non-prescription products such as vitamins and supplements make up a meaningful share of everything being taken [SRC-0007]. Each additional item adds another opportunity for two things to interact, or for two things to push in the same unwanted direction at once.

That is why the question "is this safe?" behaves so differently for an older adult who is in active cancer treatment and taking eight medicines than it does for a healthy forty-year-old. It is not that the older person is fragile. It is that the question has more moving parts, and answering it honestly requires knowing what those parts are.

There is a second reason this angle matters. When somebody proposes taking an unproven compound alongside conventional cancer treatment, the honest questions multiply. Does anything actually interact? Do the side effects overlap even without a known interaction? What is genuinely unknown, as opposed to merely unstudied in this exact situation? Those are the questions this book takes seriously, and they are the ones most viral protocols never mention.

WHAT THIS BOOK IS, AND WHAT IT IS NOT

This book will help you	This book will not do
Tell the three compounds apart and keep their evidence separate	Give a dose, schedule, cycle, or protocol of any kind
Recognize what a laboratory study, an animal study, a case report, and a clinical trial can each establish	Tell you where to obtain any product, or which product to obtain
Judge whether a study actually supports the claim being made about it	Recommend a treatment, or tell you what to take
Understand why a compelling personal story is worth attention but is not proof	Promise recovery, remission, tumor response, or survival
See why age and multiple medicines change the safety questions	Assume you are frail, confused, or unable to decide for yourself
Turn a vague online claim into a specific question for your oncology team	Provide a script for pressuring a clinician into prescribing something
Check whether a paper has been corrected, questioned, or withdrawn	Suggest that anyone is hiding a cure from you
Describe what remains genuinely unknown, and say so plainly	Pretend that uncertainty is the same as impossibility

Notice what is on the right-hand side. This book examines protocols; it does not supply them. Those are different activities, and the difference is not a formality. Explaining why a claim about a drug rests on weak evidence requires discussing the drug. Telling you how much to take, how often, and where to buy it would require pretending to a level of knowledge that does not exist for any of these compounds in cancer care. No disclaimer would repair that, so this book does not attempt it.

THE CLAIM CHECK

Running through everything that follows is a single method. It has five steps, it takes a few minutes, and it works on any claim of this kind, not just the three drugs in this book. This book will call it the Claim Check.

- **Step one: name the exact claim.** Not the mood of the video and not the general impression it left. The actual assertion. "It cures cancer" is not a claim you can check. "This compound shrank tumors in patients with this specific cancer" is.
- **Step two: name the exact compound and context.** Which of the three drugs is being discussed? A human medicine or a veterinary product? Alone, or alongside chemotherapy, radiation, or immunotherapy? For a few days, or for many months? These details are frequently missing from the claim, and their absence is itself informative.
- **Step three: identify the evidence setting.** Where did the finding come from? Cells in a dish, animals, one person's account, a database of patient records, or a controlled trial in people? Each of these answers a different question, and no one of them can substitute for another.
- **Step four: identify what is known, what is uncertain, and what is missing.** Most claims of this type contain all three at once. Separating them is most of the work, and doing so produces something far more useful than "nobody knows."
- **Step five: turn the claim into a precise question for the oncology team.** This is the step that converts reading into action. "What do you think about fenbendazole?" invites a shrug. A specific question about a specific study, a specific compound, and your specific treatment situation invites a real answer.

The Claim Check does not decide anything medical. It will not tell you whether to take something, and it is not designed to. What it does is replace a vague feeling of "there might be something to this" with an accurate account of what the evidence can and cannot carry. Chapter 1 develops each step in detail and gives you the vocabulary the steps require.

HOW THIS BOOK IS ORGANIZED

Chapter 1 teaches evidence itself. What can a cell study show? What does an animal result predict, and how often does it fail to? Why does a single trial phase mean something quite specific? How do you check whether a paper you are reading has since been corrected or withdrawn? These are the tools; the rest of the book uses them.

Chapter 2 applies those tools to fenbendazole, which is the compound at the center of most of these conversations. It covers what the drug is, why researchers became interested, what has been observed in the laboratory, what human evidence has and has not been identified, and how to think about the widely shared personal account that started much of the current wave.

Chapter 3 turns to ivermectin and mebendazole. Both have been studied in humans in cancer settings, which makes them a more complicated story than fenbendazole, not a simpler one. This chapter compares all three compounds directly and shows why evidence about one cannot be transferred to another.

Chapter 4 is the heart of the book for older readers. It examines why "is it safe?" is an incomplete question until the compound, the formulation, the duration, the person, the cancer treatment, and everything else being taken are all specified.

Chapter 5 brings all of it into the exam room. It shows how to preserve a claim and its original source, organize a complete medication picture, ask questions that get useful answers, and understand what a second opinion or a clinical trial listing can and cannot offer.

The **conclusion** and **appendices** give you the method in portable form, including printable worksheets you can take to an appointment.

UNCERTAINTY CAN BE MADE MORE PRECISE

There is a temptation, when a subject is contested, to land on one of two comfortable positions. The first is that a hidden cure is being suppressed. The second is that there is nothing here at all and anyone asking about it has been fooled.

Both positions are comfortable because both remove the need to think further. Neither is accurate, and neither serves you.

The accurate position is narrower and more useful. Real scientists have found real laboratory activity worth investigating. Some human research exists for some of these compounds. That research answers specific, limited questions, and it has not established that any of these drugs treats cancer in people.

Certain safety questions have been studied; others have not been studied at all in the situation you may be asking about.

That is not a comfortable summary. It is a precise one, and precision is what lets you act. "Nobody knows anything" leaves you nowhere. "This particular study was small, was not controlled, involved a different compound than the one being discussed, and measured something other than survival" gives you a question you can actually bring to your oncologist.

Before you can judge any protocol, you need to know what different kinds of evidence are capable of showing. That is where Chapter 1 begins.

CHAPTER 1
BEFORE YOU TRUST AN ONLINE PROTOCOL

TAKING THE CLAIM APART FROM THE STORY AROUND IT

Almost every protocol claim you will encounter arrives wrapped in a story, and the wrapping is usually better made than the contents.

The wrapping has a person in it. It has a diagnosis, a timeline, and an outcome. It may have a photograph, a scan, or a date. Somewhere inside all of that sits the actual assertion, which is a much smaller and much plainer thing. Separating the two is the first skill this chapter will teach you, because until they are separated there is nothing to evaluate. You cannot check a feeling of hope. You can check a statement.

Consider the difference between these two sentences. The first is a story: a man was told he had months to live, started taking something inexpensive, and is alive years later. The second is a claim: this compound produced tumor shrinkage in people with this type of cancer. The first sentence may be entirely true and still tell you nothing about whether the second is. They are not the same kind of statement, and only one of them can be tested.

Most viral protocol content also does something else worth noticing. It compresses. A single post may fold together a laboratory finding, a personal account, a registry listing, and a regulatory fact into one continuous paragraph, so that they appear to support each other. They usually do not. They are separate pieces of information doing separate jobs, and the compression is what makes the whole thing feel more solid than any individual part.

So the first move is mechanical. Write the claim down as one sentence, in your own words, with no story attached. Then check whether that sentence contains the four things it needs in order to be checkable: a specific compound, a specific situation, a specific outcome, and some indication of where the finding came from. Most claims are missing at least two of the four. That absence is not a small flaw. It is often the whole reason the claim sounds impressive.

There is a habit here that pays off later, and it is worth adopting from the beginning. Save the original. Take a screenshot of the post, copy the video link, note the date you found it. Claims mutate as they travel. The version you read today may have already lost the qualification that the original author included, and if you cannot get back to the source, you cannot check it. If you are researching on behalf of a family member, this is one of the most useful things you can do for them. Arriving at an appointment with a specific source is a completely different conversation from arriving with a recollection of something seen online.

WHEN SOMETHING LOOKS LIKE EVIDENCE BUT IS NOT

Protocol content has become considerably more sophisticated than it used to be. The crude version was easy to dismiss. The current version comes with charts, reference lists, molecular diagrams, and often a person in a white coat explaining it calmly. This is a real problem, because most of us learned to judge reliability by exactly those signals.

They are not reliable signals, and it is worth understanding why.

A **reference list** demonstrates that papers exist. It does not demonstrate that those papers say what the person citing them claims. This is the most common failure in the entire genre, and it is nearly always invisible unless you open the sources. A claim about a compound's effect on a particular cancer may be supported by a footnote to a real, respectable, correctly cited paper that studied a different compound, or a different cancer, or cells rather than patients. Nothing about the citation looks wrong. The number is there, the paper is real, the journal is genuine. Only the connection between the claim and the source has failed, and the only way to see it is to look.

A **chart** is a presentation choice. Any set of numbers can be drawn as a rising line. A graph showing cell death against concentration is a truthful representation of a laboratory experiment and tells you nothing about a person.

A **credential** describes the speaker, not the claim. A qualified physician making an unsupported statement is making an unsupported statement, and expertise in one area does not transfer to another. This cuts in both directions: the absence of a credential does not make someone wrong either. What matters is whether the specific assertion is supported, and that question is answered by the evidence, not by the person delivering it.

Technical vocabulary is the easiest of all to produce. Naming a pathway, a receptor, or a cellular process makes an explanation sound mechanistic, and a mechanistic explanation feels more like proof than it is. Recall that the mechanistic hypothesis sits on the bottom rung of the ladder. It is a reason to investigate, not a result.

Two further signals deserve attention because they indicate something about motive rather than content. The first is a **commercial connection**: a link to buy a product, an affiliate arrangement, a paid membership, a consultation fee. A financial interest does not make a claim false, but it does tell you the person has a reason to want you convinced, and it is a reason to check more carefully rather than less. The second is a **structural claim about suppression**, the argument that the evidence is hidden, ignored, or buried. This deserves care, because it is unfalsifiable by design. If the absence of supporting evidence is itself presented as proof that the evidence is being concealed, then no finding could ever count against the claim, and the argument has stopped being about evidence at all.

None of this means you should distrust everything that looks professional. It means the polish is not the evidence. The evidence is what the underlying sources actually establish, and that has to be checked directly.

THE EVIDENCE LADDER AND WHAT EACH RUNG CAN ANSWER

Once you have a claim, the next question is where its support came from. This matters more than almost anything else, because different kinds of research are built to answer different questions, and a finding cannot be promoted from one kind to another by being repeated.

It helps to picture a ladder. At the bottom are ideas about how something might work. Above that are experiments in cells, then in animals, then in individual people, then in groups of people, then in carefully designed trials that compare one thing against another. Each rung supports a narrower and more confident kind of statement than the rung below it.

Notice what the ladder does not say. It does not say that the lower rungs are worthless or that the people working on them are wasting their time. The lower rungs are where every treatment in existence began. What the ladder says is that a finding on one rung cannot do the work of a finding on a higher rung. A cell study cannot tell you what happens in a person, no matter how many times it is cited.

Here is the ladder in full.

Evidence type	Main question it answers	What it may show	What it cannot establish by itself
Mechanistic hypothesis	Is there a reason to think this could work?	A biological pathway worth testing	That the pathway works this way in a living person
Cell study	Does this affect cancer cells in a dish?	Activity at measurable concentrations in a dish	That this happens in a body, or at reachable exposures
Animal study	Does this affect tumors in a living organism?	Effects in a whole system, plus early safety signals	That humans respond the same way
Case report	What happened to one person?	A detailed, documented individual course	That the compound caused the outcome
Case series	Did something similar happen to several people?	A pattern worth investigating	Cause, frequency, or how many did not improve
Observational study	What happened to a group that took it?	Associations between exposure and outcome	Cause: the groups may differ in other ways
Early clinical study	Can people take it, and at what exposures?	Tolerability, exposure, and preliminary signals	Whether it helps patients live longer or better

Evidence type	Main question it answers	What it may show	What it cannot establish by itself
Mid-stage trial	Does the expected effect appear in patients?	Whether a signal is worth testing at scale	Benefit compared with standard treatment
Comparative trial	Is this better than the alternative?	Benefit or absence of benefit against a comparator	Results in populations that were not studied
Regulatory information	What has a regulator reviewed and authorized?	Approved uses, warnings, and known interactions	Anything about a use that was never reviewed

Keep this table nearby. Most of the work in evaluating a protocol claim consists of locating the claim's evidence on this ladder and then noticing that the claim was written as though it belonged several rungs higher.

Locating it is usually straightforward once you know what to look for. Words like *cells*, *cell line*, *in vitro*, and *culture* place a finding on the second rung. *Mice*, *rats*, *xenograft*, and *in vivo* place it on the third. A named individual places it on the fourth. *Cohort*, *registry*, *retrospective*, and *records* indicate the sixth. *Phase* followed by a number places it in the clinical rungs, and the number tells you which question was being asked. If none of these words appear anywhere in the claim or its sources, you have not yet found where the evidence came from, and that is the next thing to establish rather than a detail to move past.

There is one more piece of language to get right, because it is the source of a great deal of unnecessary argument. When someone reports that no study exists, what they can honestly mean is that no study was found in a particular search, of particular databases and registries, on a particular date, for a particular kind of study. That is a real and useful finding, and it should be stated with those limits attached. It is a different statement from "no such study exists anywhere," which almost nobody is in a position to make. The same discipline applies in the other direction. "No known interaction" means nobody has documented one, which is not the same as evidence that two things do not interact. It frequently means the question has not been studied.

This distinction is not pedantry. Whole arguments online consist of one side saying there is no evidence and the other saying the evidence is being suppressed, when the accurate statement is narrower and available to both: a specific search, on a specific date, found a specific amount of a specific kind of evidence. That sentence can be checked. The other two cannot.

WHY LABORATORY PLAUSIBILITY IS NOT A CLINICAL OUTCOME

The single most common move in protocol content is to present a cell-culture or animal finding as though it were a patient result. It usually is not done dishonestly. It happens because the laboratory language sounds like the clinical language. "Killed cancer cells" and "treated cancer" use similar words for entirely different events.

Three things go wrong on the way from a dish to a person, and understanding them will let you spot the gap yourself.

The first is exposure. In a laboratory, researchers decide the concentration around the cells and hold it there. In a person, the amount that reaches a tumor depends on how much is absorbed from the gut, how quickly the liver processes it, how it distributes through tissue, and how fast it is cleared. Some compounds simply cannot reach, in a living body, the concentrations at which they were active in a dish. That is not a technicality. It can be the entire explanation for why a promising laboratory result goes nowhere.

The second is context. Cancer cells in a dish sit in a uniform environment with no blood supply, no immune system, no surrounding tissue, and no other organs to protect. A tumor in a person sits inside a system that is far more complicated and that pushes back in ways a dish cannot reproduce.

The third is that living systems have more ways to be harmed. A compound that damages cancer cells may damage other cells too. In a dish, nobody is measuring what happens to the liver.

This is why the numbers on translation are as sobering as they are. When researchers examined tens of thousands of drug development programs that had already progressed far enough to enter human testing, the overall probability of eventually reaching approval was under fifteen percent, and cancer programs had the lowest rate of any major category [SRC-0010]. These were not casual ideas. Each had already survived laboratory and animal work convincing enough to justify testing in people, and most still did not arrive.

That statistic is worth sitting with, because it cuts in both directions. It explains why a laboratory finding, however striking, is not a reason to expect benefit. It also explains why the failure of one compound is not evidence of a conspiracy. Most candidates fail. That is the ordinary condition of drug development, not a sign that something has gone wrong.

WHY AN ANECDOTE CAN MATTER WITHOUT PROVING ANYTHING

There is a way of dismissing personal accounts that is both common and wrong. It treats anyone who reports an unexpected recovery as either mistaken or lying. That posture is unkind, and it is also bad reasoning. Unusual things do happen, people do report them accurately, and some genuine discoveries have started exactly this way.

The honest position is different. A personal account can be completely true and still not establish what caused the outcome.

Suppose someone with advanced cancer began taking a compound and is doing well two years later. Every part of that may be documented. The question that remains is why, and there are several answers competing for the same evidence. The person may have been receiving conventional treatment at the same time, which is very often the case. The cancer may have been a type or subtype with a better outlook than the initial conversation suggested. The initial prognosis may have been a population average rather than a prediction about this individual. Other things may have changed at the same time. And in rare cases, cancers do behave unexpectedly for reasons nobody yet understands.

None of those possibilities is dismissive. All of them are live, and a single account cannot distinguish between them.

There is a further problem, and it has nothing to do with the honesty of any individual. You are not seeing a representative sample. People who take something and do well are far more likely to post about it than people who take the same thing and do not. Nobody films an update to report that nothing happened. So the accounts that reach you have already been filtered, and the filter selects precisely for the outcome that makes the claim look strongest. This is not a criticism of the people posting. It is a description of what any collection of volunteered stories will look like.

When a report is written up formally by clinicians, with dates, imaging, pathology, and concurrent treatment documented, it becomes a **case report**, and it moves up the ladder. A well-written case report is genuinely valuable. It is precise about what was observed and honest about what it cannot explain, and it often generates the research question that a trial later answers. What it still cannot do is establish cause, or tell you how often the same thing happens.

Several such reports collected together form a **case series**. A series is more informative than a single report, because a repeated pattern is harder to explain as coincidence. It carries the same fundamental limit, though, and adds one of its own: nobody knows how many people had the same exposure without the same result, because those people were never written up. A series of ten favorable cases might represent ten out of twelve, or ten out of ten thousand. From the series alone, there is no way to tell.

This is worth stating positively, because the point is easily mistaken for dismissal. Personal accounts are how a great many research questions begin. A clinician notices something unexpected, writes it up carefully, another clinician recognizes the pattern, and eventually somebody designs a study to find out whether the pattern is real. That pathway is legitimate and it has produced genuine discoveries. What the pathway requires is the study at the end of it. A story is the beginning of the process, and treating it as the conclusion skips the part where we find out whether it was true.

APPROVED, OFF-LABEL, INVESTIGATIONAL, VETERINARY

Four words get used interchangeably in protocol discussions, and they mean four different things. Getting them straight will resolve a surprising number of arguments.

Approved means a regulator reviewed evidence and authorized a specific use. Approval is always tied to an indication, a population, and a set of conditions described on the label. It carries a finding that, for that use, the benefits were judged to outweigh the risks. It carries no finding at all about any other use.

Off-label describes a clinician prescribing an approved drug for a use the regulator has not reviewed. This is legal and often appropriate. A clinician may do it because no approved treatment exists for a condition, or because approved options have been exhausted. The regulator's own patient guidance is explicit that in this situation the agency has not determined that the drug is safe and effective for that unapproved use [SRC-0011]. That sentence is worth reading twice. Off-label use is not a loophole that quietly extends approval; it is a decision made by a clinician, for one patient, in the absence of regulatory review.

Investigational means a compound is being studied under a formal research plan, with oversight, documented consent, defined endpoints, and monitoring. A drug under investigation for a cancer indication has not been shown to work for it. That is the reason the study exists.

Veterinary means approved for animals, with dosing and safety established for a species that is not you. It says nothing about human suitability in either direction.

Now notice how these get blended online. "It is approved for humans" becomes "it is safe." "Doctors prescribe things off-label all the time" becomes "so this is normal practice." "There is a trial running" becomes "the experts already know it works." Each of those is a promotion the evidence has not earned, and each is easy to catch once you have the four words separated.

One more distinction belongs here, and it is the one most often skipped. Two products can contain the same active compound and still be different things in practice. **Formulation** governs how much of a compound is absorbed, how quickly, and how consistently. It covers the physical form, the substances the compound is mixed with, the manufacturing standards applied, and the testing done to confirm that each unit contains what the label says. A product made under human pharmaceutical standards and a product made for another purpose may share an active ingredient and differ substantially in everything else.

This is why the phrase "the same drug" does so much unearned work in protocol content. A study conducted with a pharmaceutical-grade preparation, at a known exposure, in supervised conditions, is not evidence about a different preparation taken differently. When you read a claim, formulation belongs alongside compound, exposure, duration, and combination context as one of the details that has to be pinned down before the claim means anything specific.

One further point. Self-administering a compound outside medical care is none of the four categories above. It is not approval, it is not off-label prescribing, it is not investigational research, and adding a supplement schedule or a blood test does not convert it into any of them. Whatever else it may be, it is not a category that carries the protections those words describe.

READING A TRIAL FOR WHAT IT ACTUALLY MEASURED

Clinical trials are where most protocol arguments end up, and they are also where the most confident misreadings happen. You do not need a research degree to read a trial usefully. You need to ask what it was built to find out.

Human studies are conventionally described in phases. The regulator's own description is a good place to start: early studies typically involve twenty to eighty people, mid-stage studies from a few dozen to around three hundred, and late-stage studies from several hundred to around three thousand [SRC-0009].

Those numbers matter, but the purpose behind them matters more.

A **Phase I** study is asking whether people can take a compound and what happens to it in the body at different exposures. It is a safety and feasibility study. Some Phase I studies in cancer do report tumor measurements, and those observations are worth having, but the study was not built to determine whether the compound helps, and it usually has no comparison group at all.

A **Phase II** study asks whether the effect people are hoping for shows up in patients at a rate that justifies a larger investment. Some Phase II studies have a comparison group and some do not.

A **Phase III** study asks the question most readers care about: is this better than the alternative? These are the studies that support approval, and they are built around comparison.

Within any of these, a handful of design features determine what the results can carry.

An **endpoint** is the thing the study measured. This is the detail most often lost in translation. A study measuring tumor shrinkage and a study measuring survival are answering different questions, and a compound can improve one without improving the other. When a claim says something "worked," your next question is always: measured how?

A **predefined benchmark** is the result the researchers committed to in advance as the threshold for success. Committing beforehand matters, because any dataset examined long enough will produce something that looks interesting. A result that clears a benchmark set in advance is much stronger than an interesting pattern noticed afterward.

A **control** or **comparator** is what the treatment group is measured against, whether an inactive placebo, the current standard treatment, or no additional treatment. Without one, you know what happened to the people who took the compound, but not what would have happened otherwise.

Randomization is assigning participants to groups by chance rather than by choice. Its purpose is to make the groups comparable in ways nobody thought to measure. It is the single most powerful tool for making a comparison trustworthy.

Blinding means participants, clinicians, or assessors do not know who received what, so expectations cannot influence how outcomes are reported. It is valuable where feasible, and it is not always possible. Some interventions cannot be disguised, and the absence of blinding is a limitation to weigh rather than an automatic disqualification.

Sample size governs what a study can detect. A small study that finds nothing has not shown that nothing is there. A small study that finds something dramatic may be reporting an unusual result. Neither conclusion follows automatically from the number of participants, but the number tells you how much weight the result can bear.

Selection bias occurs when the people in a study differ systematically from those who are not, in ways that affect the outcome. If a compound is taken mainly by people who are healthier, more mobile, or more engaged with their care, their outcomes may reflect those characteristics rather than the compound.

Confounding is the more general version of the same problem. Something other than the treatment differs between the groups and influences the result. Randomization exists to address confounding; observational studies must attempt to adjust for it statistically, which helps but never fully settles the question.

A **surrogate outcome** is a measurement used as a stand-in for the outcome people actually care about, chosen because it can be observed sooner. Tumor shrinkage standing in for survival is the familiar example in cancer. Regulators distinguish carefully between surrogates validated by clinical data showing they predict real benefit and those merely thought likely to [SRC-0012, SRC-0013]. In protocol content, surrogate results are routinely reported as though they were the real thing.

An **observational study** watches what happens without assigning treatment. It can cover far more people than a trial and can detect patterns worth investigating. What it cannot do is establish cause, because the people who chose the exposure differ from those who did not in ways no statistical adjustment fully removes.

Two words that appear constantly in protocol discussions deserve separate handling, because both are routinely stretched past what they can bear.

The first is **signal**. In research, a signal is an observation suggestive enough to justify a further study, and no more. A few tumors that shrank in an early trial with no comparison group constitute a signal. So does a pattern noticed in a database. Signals are how research decides what to investigate next, which makes them genuinely important. What a signal is not is a conclusion. When a claim describes something as promising, encouraging, or showing potential, it is usually describing a signal, and the honest translation is that somebody thinks this is worth another study.

The second is **failure**. When a trial does not meet its predefined benchmark, this is often reported online in one of two equally wrong ways. One side treats it as proof that the whole idea was worthless. The other treats it as proof of nothing at all, or of interference.

Neither reading is right, and the accurate one is more informative than both. A trial that misses its benchmark has answered a specific question about a specific compound, at a specific exposure, in a specific population, measured a specific way. It may mean the compound does not help. It may also mean the exposure was too low, the population was chosen poorly, the measurement was the wrong one, or the study was too small to detect a real but modest effect. A negative result does not disprove the underlying biological idea, and it certainly does not disprove the laboratory findings that prompted the trial. Those findings remain exactly what they were.

But a negative trial is also real evidence, and it counts. It is not a neutral event to be set aside while attention moves to the next favorable anecdote. When you evaluate a claim, unfavorable results deserve the same reading you would give a favorable one: what was measured, in whom, compared with what, and what does it therefore support?

WHEN MORE THAN ONE THING IS HAPPENING AT ONCE

A specific attribution problem deserves its own section, because it appears in nearly every protocol account and is almost never acknowledged.

Very few people take an unproven compound and nothing else. Most are also receiving conventional treatment, often several supplements, sometimes dietary changes, sometimes a new exercise routine. When the outcome is good, the compound gets the credit, because it is the interesting part of the story.

The formal version of this problem shows up in research too. When a study tests a combination, its results describe the combination. Unless the design specifically isolates the contribution of one component, usually by including a group that received everything except that component, the study cannot tell you what any single ingredient did. A trial of chemotherapy plus a repurposed compound that shows a good outcome has shown something about the pair. It has not shown that the repurposed compound was responsible, and it has not shown that it was irrelevant either. The question was not asked.

So when you read a favorable account, the working question is not "did this person do well?" It is "what else was happening at the same time, and can anything here separate the contributions?" Frequently the honest answer is that nothing can. That answer is not a dismissal. It is an accurate description of what the available information supports.

PUBLICATION IS NOT THE FINISH LINE

Many readers treat publication in a journal as the end of the verification process. It is closer to the beginning.

Peer review means other researchers in the field read the manuscript before publication and raised objections. It is a filter, and a useful one. It is not a guarantee. Reviewers work from what the authors submitted, usually cannot inspect the underlying data, and vary widely in how thoroughly they read.

A **preprint** is a manuscript posted publicly before peer review. Preprints are legitimate and often valuable, particularly when information needs to move quickly. But a preprint has not yet been through the filter, and this should be visible in how you weigh it. Protocol content frequently cites preprints without mentioning their status.

After publication, three kinds of notice can attach to a paper, and knowing the difference is genuinely useful.

A **correction** fixes a specific error while the paper's conclusions stand.

An **expression of concern** is a notice alerting readers that credible concerns have been raised about a paper's reliability, in situations that do not meet the threshold for retraction or where conclusive evidence cannot be obtained for some time. It can be an interim step on the way to a correction or retraction, or it can be the final state of a paper that will not be resolved further [SRC-0015]. A paper carrying an expression of concern has not been withdrawn, and it has not been cleared either. Treating it as ordinary evidence misrepresents where it stands.

A **retraction** is the strongest notice. It is issued when a paper is considered so unreliable that its findings and conclusions cannot be depended upon, whether because of honest error or misconduct. Its purpose is to correct the scientific record rather than to punish anyone [SRC-0014]. A retracted paper should not be used to support a factual claim, and yet retracted work continues to circulate in protocol content long after withdrawal, often because the original post was never updated.

Checking for these notices takes a minute or two. Open the paper on the journal's own site rather than on an aggregator or a PDF someone shared. Journals display corrections, expressions of concern, and retractions on the article page, and the major biomedical databases display them alongside the record. If a source is a video or a post rather than a paper, this is exactly why you saved the original citation.

In practice the whole check is short, and it is worth walking through once so it becomes routine.

Start with the claim and find the source it names. If it names none, that is your finding, and you can stop. If it names a paper, search for the title in a biomedical database or in a general search engine, and open the version on the publisher's own site. Look first at the top of the article page, where notices appear, and at the abstract, which usually states the study type and what was measured. Two questions answer themselves almost immediately: is this the compound the claim was about, and is this cells, animals, or people?

Then read the last part of the abstract, the conclusion, and compare it with the claim you wrote down in step one. This comparison is where most protocol claims come apart, and it takes about thirty seconds. Researchers are generally careful in their conclusions. They write that something warrants further investigation, or that an effect was observed in a particular model. The claim built on top of that paper is often several rungs more confident than anything the authors wrote.

If the paper is behind a paywall, the abstract is usually free and is normally enough for this purpose. It will tell you the compound, the model, the design, and the measured outcome, which is most of what the Claim Check needs.

One more status is frequently misread. A **trial registration** is a public record that a study is planned or running. In the United States, registration in the public registry is a legal requirement for many clinical trials, triggered by the study beginning, along with an obligation to submit summary results afterward [SRC-0016]. The registration is therefore an administrative record, not a scientific verdict, and certainly not an endorsement. A registry entry tells you that someone is asking a question. It does not tell you the answer, and if the results field is empty, no answer has been posted.

THE CLAIM CHECK, EXPANDED

You met the Claim Check in the introduction. Now that you have the vocabulary, here is the working version, with the questions to ask at each step.

Step one. Name the exact claim.

What exactly is being asserted? Write it as one sentence with the story removed. If you cannot, the claim may be too vague to evaluate, which is itself a finding.

Step two. Name the exact compound and context.

Which compound, specifically? A human medicine or a veterinary product? Used alone or alongside other treatment? For days or for months? In what cancer type, at what stage? Every missing detail is a place where the claim may be borrowing credibility from something it is not describing.

Step three. Identify the evidence setting and the outcome measured.

Where on the ladder does the support sit? Then, separately: what was actually measured? Cells affected, tumors shrunk, symptoms improved, people living longer? These are different results, and the difference between the claim and the measurement is often the whole story.

Step four. Identify what is known, what is uncertain, and what is missing.

What alternative explanations remain unexcluded? Was there a comparison group? Was anything else happening at the same time? And has the source or its status changed since it was published? Most claims contain all three categories at once. Separating them is the real work.

Step five. Turn it into a precise question for the oncology team.

Convert what you have found into one specific question that a clinician can actually answer, about your situation.

A note on what this tool is and is not. Working through five steps does not entitle anyone to conclude that a compound is safe or worth taking. The Claim Check tells you what the evidence can carry. It does not tell you what to do, and no amount of careful reading replaces the clinical judgment that applies to one particular person.

WHAT THIS CHAPTER DOES NOT ASK OF YOU

Two things are worth saying plainly before moving on.

The first concerns effort. Everything in this chapter takes attention, and attention is exactly what is in short supply when someone is ill, when appointments are stacking up, and when the reading happens at the end of a long day. Under those conditions a simple, confident narrative is more appealing than a careful one, and that is true of everyone. It is not a failing of any age group. It is a predictable consequence of being tired and frightened, and the content that spreads best is built, deliberately or not, to take advantage of it. Knowing that is a defense in itself.

This is also where a family member can be most useful. Not by taking over the decision, but by holding the paperwork: keeping the original link, noting the date, writing down which compound was named, and bringing the list to the appointment. That is real work, and it does not require displacing anyone.

The second concerns standards. This book is written in plain language on purpose, and plain language is a matter of how things are explained. It is not a reduction in what counts as proof. A claim does not become better supported because it has been explained more simply, and a reader is not owed a lower standard of evidence because a book was written to be readable. Those are separate things, and conflating them would defeat the purpose of the entire exercise.

WHERE THIS LEADS

You now have a ladder, a set of design questions, a way to check whether a paper still stands, and a five-step method for working through any claim of this type.

None of it means much in the abstract. The test is whether it holds up against the most visible claim in this entire subject, the one that brought most readers here, and the one with the largest gap between how confidently it is stated online and how much evidence actually supports it.

That claim is about fenbendazole, and it is where the next chapter begins.

CHAPTER 2
FENBENDAZOLE: WHAT THE EVIDENCE ACTUALLY SHOWS

WHAT THIS COMPOUND IS

Fenbendazole is a deworming drug for animals.

That sentence is the honest starting point, and it is worth sitting with before anything else is added to it. Fenbendazole was developed as a veterinary anthelmintic and is used in cattle, horses, pigs, dogs, cats, and other species to treat roundworm, whipworm, pinworm, and hookworm infections. In the United States it is approved for those animal uses, and only those. There is no approved human formulation and no approved human indication [SRC-0017].

Chemically it belongs to the benzimidazole family, which also includes mebendazole and albendazole, both of which are approved human medicines. All of these compounds work against parasites in essentially the same way. They bind selectively to a protein called beta-tubulin in the worm, which the worm needs in order to maintain its internal structure. Disrupt that, and the parasite becomes immobilised and dies [SRC-0017].

Two features of the drug explain much of what follows. The first is that it binds parasite tubulin far more readily than it binds the equivalent protein in mammals. That selectivity is the whole reason it can be given safely to a dog. The second is that it is poorly absorbed when taken by mouth. Most of it stays in the digestive tract. That is exactly what you want when the target is an intestinal worm. It is exactly the opposite of what you would want if the target were a tumour elsewhere in the body.

Neither of those features is a criticism. They are simply what the compound is, and both become important later.

It is worth pausing on the reflex the word *veterinary* provokes. Some readers hear it and conclude that anyone interested must be desperate or foolish. Others hear the dismissal and conclude that the establishment is being snobbish about a cheap drug. Chapter 1 dealt with this: a veterinary origin says nothing either way about whether a molecule is worth studying. What matters is what has been found out. So let us find out.

WHY RESEARCHERS BECAME INTERESTED

The interest is real, and it did not come from social media. It came from a laboratory accident.

In 2008, researchers at a US institution were running an experiment using mice carrying implanted human lymphoma tumours. The mice were being given fenbendazole in their feed as a routine measure against pinworm, which is standard practice in animal facilities. The tumours failed to grow. That was not the result anyone was looking for, and it threatened to ruin the experiment [SRC-0018].

The team investigated. They discovered that the fenbendazole had been mixed into a feed that had also been supplemented with extra vitamins, and they set up a small study to work out which ingredient was responsible. Twenty mice were divided across four groups: ordinary feed, feed with added vitamins, feed with fenbendazole, and feed with both.

The result is the single most important and most consistently omitted fact in this entire subject. **Fenbendazole alone did not alter tumour growth.** Vitamins alone did not alter tumour growth. Only the combination produced a significant effect, and the authors were explicit that the mechanism of that synergy was unknown and needed investigation. Their practical conclusion was a warning to other researchers: be careful using this drug during tumour studies, because it may interact with other treatments and confound results [SRC-0018].

That is a genuinely interesting finding. It is also almost the opposite of the claim built on top of it. The paper that launched the fenbendazole story is a paper in which fenbendazole by itself did nothing.

There is a broader reason researchers find this family of compounds interesting, and it is legitimate. Microtubules, the structures built from tubulin, are essential to cell division. Several established chemotherapy drugs work by interfering with them. If a benzimidazole binds mammalian tubulin at all, even weakly, there is a mechanistic reason to ask whether it might affect rapidly dividing cells. That is a reasonable question. Chapter 1 placed it precisely: it is a mechanistic hypothesis, the bottom rung of the ladder, and it is a reason to investigate rather than a result.

It is worth saying clearly that the idea behind all of this, taking a drug developed for one purpose and testing it for another, is not fringe. It is called drug repurposing, and it is an established field with dedicated research groups, funding streams, and journals. The logic is straightforward. A compound already used in humans has a known manufacturing process, a known safety profile in its original setting, and often no remaining patent protection, which makes it cheap. If such a compound turned out to work against a cancer, it could reach patients faster and at lower cost than a new molecule.

Several widely used cancer treatments began as something else. So the proposition that an old, inexpensive, unglamorous drug might have unrecognised value is not a conspiracy theory. It is an ordinary scientific hypothesis, and researchers take it seriously.

What repurposing does not do is skip the evidence. A repurposed candidate still has to be shown to reach the target, at a workable exposure, with acceptable harms, and to actually help patients. Being repurposed is a reason a compound might be studied. It is not a reason to believe it works, and the fact that a hypothesis is reasonable tells you nothing about whether it turns out to be true.

WHAT THE LABORATORY AND ANIMAL RESEARCH HAS SHOWN

Here the story becomes genuinely mixed, and the mixture is the point.

The most frequently cited supportive study was published in 2018 in *Scientific Reports*. Working with human non-small-cell lung cancer cell lines, the researchers reported that fenbendazole showed moderate affinity for mammalian tubulin and was toxic to cancer cells at micromolar concentrations. They also reported effects on p53, a protein involved in how a cell responds to damage. And they reported interference with how the cell takes up glucose, including reduced levels of glucose transporters and of a key enzyme the cell uses to burn it. In mice carrying human tumour grafts, orally administered fenbendazole inhibited tumour growth [SRC-0020].

That is a real finding in a real journal, and it should not be waved away. It is also worth reading exactly as written. The authors described the compound as a *moderate* microtubule destabilising agent, not a potent one. The cell activity occurred at micromolar concentrations. That is a specific quantity of drug around the cells, and Chapter 1 explained why the number matters. Whether a dish responds at that concentration is one question. Whether a living body can reach and hold that concentration at a tumour is a completely different one.

Now the study that protocol content rarely mentions.

In 2013, a group at Yale set out to test fenbendazole properly as an anti-cancer agent, using a mouse mammary tumour line both in culture and as solid tumours in living mice. In culture, intensive treatment was toxic to the cells, with toxicity increasing with longer exposure and under low-oxygen conditions. That part is consistent with the other laboratory work.

Then they tested it in animals. Fenbendazole, given in what the authors described as maximally intensive regimens, did not alter the growth of the tumours. It did not increase the effect of radiation. Combined with a taxane chemotherapy drug, it produced simply additive toxicity rather than any synergy. Their conclusion was unambiguous: these studies provided no evidence that fenbendazole would have value in cancer therapy, although the wider class of compounds merited further investigation [SRC-0019].

So the animal picture is not one-directional. One study found tumour inhibition in one model. Another study, specifically designed to look for it, found none in a different model. A third found an effect only in combination with something else. This is what an unresolved preclinical question actually looks like, and it is very different from the impression given by a video that cites only the favourable result.

None of this makes the supportive findings fraudulent, and none of it makes the negative findings decisive. Different tumour models behave differently, and a compound can be active against one cancer type and inert against another. That is precisely why the question cannot be settled in mice, and why the disagreement between these studies is an argument for human trials rather than a substitute for them.

Two features of this literature are worth understanding, because they affect how much weight the whole body of work can bear.

The first concerns what these mouse experiments actually are. The usual method is called a xenograft. Human cancer cells are grown in culture, then implanted into mice, often just under the skin. The mice have had their immune systems disabled, so that the human tissue is not rejected. This is a useful tool and it has contributed to real discoveries. It is also a long way from a person with cancer. The tumour is in the wrong place. It did not arise naturally. It has not developed the internal variety that real tumours accumulate over years. And it sits in an animal with no working immune system. That last point matters a great deal. The immune system is one of the most important participants in how cancers behave, and many modern treatments work through it. A compound that shrinks a lump under the skin of an immune-deficient mouse has demonstrated something. It has not demonstrated what it would do in a person.

The second is a problem with the published record itself. Experiments that find an effect are considerably more likely to be written up and published than experiments that find nothing. A researcher who tests a compound and sees no result often has little incentive to prepare a manuscript, and journals have historically been less interested in publishing one. The practical consequence is that the visible literature on any compound tends to look more favourable than the complete set of experiments actually performed. This is a recognised issue across biomedical research and it is not specific to fenbendazole. But it means that when you count the supportive papers, you are counting what was published rather than what was found. The Yale study is a useful reminder. Negative results do exist, when someone takes the trouble to report them.

WHY THE GAP TO HUMANS IS ESPECIALLY WIDE HERE

Chapter 1 described three reasons laboratory findings fail to reach patients: exposure, context, and harm. For fenbendazole, the first of these is not a general caution. It is a specific, well-documented problem.

Fenbendazole is poorly absorbed from the gut. This is a designed feature, and it is why the drug works well against intestinal worms in animals. What is absorbed is rapidly processed by the liver into other compounds, principally one called oxfendazole, along with further metabolites, through enzyme systems that also handle a great many prescription medicines [SRC-0027].

Put those two facts together and a difficult question emerges. If very little of the compound crosses into the bloodstream, and what does cross is quickly converted into something else, what concentration actually reaches a tumour in a person? The honest answer as of this book's research cutoff is that nobody knows, because the pharmacokinetics of fenbendazole in humans have not been properly characterised. There is no approved human formulation, so there has been no regulatory requirement to establish this, and the published literature does not fill the gap [SRC-0017, SRC-0027].

This is not a small technical footnote. Everything about the laboratory case for fenbendazole depends on cancer cells being exposed to a certain concentration of drug. If that concentration cannot be achieved or sustained in a human being, the laboratory findings do not transfer, however elegant the mechanism.

And the one thing we can say with confidence is that the question has not been answered.

The metabolism point matters in a second way as well. A compound handled by the same liver enzyme systems as many prescription drugs is a compound with a real potential for interactions. What that means for someone in cancer treatment is a Chapter 4 question, and it is taken up there.

There is one indirect source of human information, and it is genuinely relevant. Fenbendazole is converted in the body into a compound called oxfendazole, which is its principal active metabolite. Oxfendazole has been developed in its own right as a possible human antiparasitic treatment. It has been through a first-in-human study in healthy volunteers, looking at what the body does with it and how well it is tolerated [SRC-0028].

Two things follow from that, pulling in opposite directions.

The first is that this is the closest thing to human pharmacokinetic data that exists in this area, and it exists because someone did the proper work on a related compound. It is a demonstration that these studies are entirely possible to run.

The second is what that study observed. Liver enzyme abnormalities were among the findings [SRC-0022, SRC-0028]. That is a signal, in Chapter 1's sense of the word, and it points in the same direction as the human case reports discussed later in this chapter.

It would be a mistake to treat oxfendazole data as though it were fenbendazole data. They are different compounds, studied in healthy volunteers rather than cancer patients, at exposures established for a different purpose. Chapter 1's rule against transferring evidence between compounds applies here as much as anywhere. What the oxfendazole work does establish is narrower, and still useful. The questions are answerable and the methods exist. And where a benzimidazole metabolite has been examined carefully in people, the liver is where attention has landed.

WHAT HUMAN EVIDENCE EXISTS

This section is short, and its shortness is the finding.

As of this book's research cutoff, a search of the published literature and of the public trial registry identifies no completed clinical trial of fenbendazole as a cancer treatment in humans. No Phase I study establishing what happens to it in the body of a cancer patient. No Phase II study looking for a signal. No comparative trial. The US government maintains an authoritative resource on drug-induced liver injury. It keeps a monograph on fenbendazole, precisely because the compound is being used off label. That monograph states plainly that fenbendazole has not been shown to be effective in treating any form of cancer in humans [SRC-0017].

In May 2026, the American Society of Clinical Oncology issued a clinical notice on this subject. Its position is direct. There is no robust, peer-reviewed clinical evidence that fenbendazole is safe or effective for treating any human cancer. Well-designed comparative trials would be needed to establish whether it has any benefit worth the harms [SRC-0026].

Note the shape of that statement, because Chapter 1 insisted on this distinction. It is not a claim that fenbendazole has been proven useless. It is a statement that the study which would settle the question has not been done.

It is also worth being precise about the limits of the search behind this section, in exactly the way Chapter 1 recommended. Here is the statement with its limits attached. As of July 2026, a search of the published biomedical literature and of the public US trial registry did not identify a completed clinical trial of fenbendazole as a cancer treatment in humans. Authoritative reviews and a major oncology society describe the same absence. That is a bounded finding with a date attached. It is not a claim that no such study exists anywhere in the world. If one is completed and published after this book goes to press, the right response is to read it. Not to defend the sentence you are reading now.

There is a second thing you will encounter online that resembles human evidence and is not. Websites and social media groups maintain running compilations of self-reported cases, sometimes numbering in the hundreds. These are presented, and often described, as case series.

They are not. A case series, in the medical sense, is a set of individual patients documented by clinicians. Their diagnoses, treatments, imaging, and outcomes are recorded, and reported in enough detail that another clinician can evaluate them. A compilation of volunteered online reports has none of that. There is usually no confirmation that the diagnosis was what the person believed it was. There is no record of what conventional treatment was running at the same time. There is no imaging. And there is no follow-up on anyone who stopped posting. Above all, there is no denominator: nobody knows how many people took the compound and did not improve, because those people did not write in.

The number is doing the persuasive work. Three hundred reports feels overwhelming compared with three published cases. But three hundred unverified accounts, collected by self-selection, do not add up to more evidence than three documented ones. They add up to a different kind of thing entirely. No quantity of them will ever convert into the other kind.

What does exist in the human literature is a small number of individual case reports, and those are worth examining carefully, because they include both of the things the internet reports selectively.

THE ACCOUNT THAT STARTED THIS

Almost every reader of this book has encountered some version of one particular story. Rather than retell it as inspiration, this section will do what Chapter 1 trained you to do: separate what is documented from what is inferred.

The documented facts are not in dispute. In 2016 a man in Oklahoma was diagnosed with small-cell lung cancer that had spread widely. The prognosis he was given was measured in months. He received care at a major US cancer centre and enrolled in a clinical trial of pembrolizumab, an immunotherapy drug. Separately, and on his own initiative, he began taking fenbendazole along with several supplements. Some months later, imaging showed no detectable cancer. He has remained well for years since, and he has said openly and consistently that he took both things at once [SRC-0027].

Now apply step four of the Claim Check: what is known, what is uncertain, what is missing?

What is known is that a man with a very poor prognosis experienced a dramatic and durable remission. There is no reason to doubt that, and it would be both unkind and unjustified to suggest otherwise.

What is uncertain is why. He was receiving pembrolizumab, an approved immunotherapy that produces durable remissions in a subset of patients and that was, at the time, in a clinical trial precisely because its effects were being studied. He was also taking fenbendazole and supplements. This is the co-intervention problem from Chapter 1 in its purest form. One person, two or more simultaneous interventions, one outcome, and no way to attribute it. That is not a criticism of him. It is a structural feature of the situation, and it would apply equally to any individual case.

A frequently repeated element of the account is that he was the only patient in a large trial cohort to respond this way. Medical privacy makes that claim impossible for anyone outside the trial to verify, and it should therefore be held loosely rather than treated as established. The claim is also often used as though it ruled out the immunotherapy. It does not. A single exceptional responder within a trial is a well-recognised phenomenon in cancer medicine. It is precisely the sort of case that trials exist to find.

Here is the most important thing to understand about this account, and it applies regardless of what actually caused the remission. Even if fenbendazole contributed, a single case cannot tell you how often that happens, in whom, with which cancers, at what exposure, or at what cost. Chapter 1 made this point about case reports generally. It applies here with full force, and it would apply with equal force if the account were about a pharmaceutical company's drug.

Finally, notice what has grown around the account since. What began as one man's description of his own experience has become a named protocol, a genre of video, a network of commercial sellers, and a body of compiled testimonials. Almost none of that additional structure was generated by evidence. It was generated by attention.

This matters for a practical reason. The man at the centre of the story has, by all appearances, been sincere and has consistently acknowledged that he was receiving immunotherapy at the same time. The ecosystem built on top of his account has not always been so careful. Search for the protocol today and you will find pages that present it as established. Many omit the immunotherapy entirely. Many describe the outcome as proof. And many offer to sell you the compound before you have finished reading.

That last feature is worth dwelling on. A page that reports a claim and a page that sells the product behind it are doing different jobs. Chapter 1 identified a commercial connection as a reason to check more carefully, not less. A great deal of the material a worried reader will encounter on this subject is not journalism, is not research, and is not one patient talking to another. It is retail, and its purpose is not to help you evaluate the evidence.

None of that reflects on the original account, and none of it is a reason to be dismissive of the man who told it. It is a reason to notice that the story you are reading has usually passed through several hands since he told it, and that some of those hands had an interest in what you concluded.

WHAT THE PUBLISHED CASE REPORTS SHOW

Beyond that account, a handful of individual cases involving fenbendazole have been formally published. They fall into two groups, and the internet reliably reports one of them.

The favourable reports. A small number of case reports have described tumour reduction in patients who were self-administering fenbendazole. The most prominent of these was a 2025 case series in *Case Reports in Oncology* describing three patients with stage IV cancers who experienced complete or near-complete responses [SRC-0024].

That paper was retracted on 21 January 2026 [SRC-0025].

The reason matters, and it should be stated precisely rather than weaponised in either direction. The retraction notice states that concerns were raised after publication about an undeclared conflict of interest. At the time of submission, the first author was offering services related to the subject of the study. This was not disclosed in the paper's conflict-of-interest statement. The journal contacted the author, found the response unsatisfactory, and concluded that the omission would have affected how the work should be interpreted [SRC-0025].

So the retraction was not a finding that the clinical data were fabricated. It was a finding that a material financial interest was concealed from readers who were entitled to know about it when weighing the authors' interpretation. Chapter 1 explained what that status means in practice: a retracted paper should not be used to support a factual claim. It has been withdrawn from the scientific record. That remains true whether or not the underlying observations were accurate, and it is not altered by anyone's opinion about why the retraction happened.

This is also a live demonstration of why the publication-status check exists. That paper circulated for months as the most-cited piece of clinical literature in fenbendazole discussion. Anyone who saved the citation and checked it later would have found the notice. Anyone relying on a video from 2025 would not.

The harm reports. The other group is larger, more recent, and more consistent.

Several published cases describe clinically apparent liver injury in people taking fenbendazole for cancer on their own initiative. In 2021, an 80-year-old woman with advanced lung cancer was receiving pembrolizumab. About a month after starting fenbendazole on her own, she developed severe liver injury. Her liver function recovered once she stopped it, and she was able to continue her immunotherapy. Her tumour did not shrink [SRC-0021]. In 2024, a 67-year-old woman developed jaundice and fatigue after about a year of self-administration. Her liver enzymes were many times the upper limit of normal. This was the first case confirmed by examining liver tissue. Her liver tests returned to normal three months after she stopped [SRC-0022]. In 2026, a 47-year-old woman with metastatic colon cancer was on immunotherapy. She developed liver injury weeks after starting fenbendazole and then increasing it. She recovered after stopping, and was later able to resume her cancer treatment [SRC-0023]. Further cases have been reported, including in a patient with pre-existing cirrhosis.

The US government's LiverTox resource, updated in April 2026, assigns fenbendazole a likelihood score of C, meaning a probable cause of clinically apparent liver injury. The same source notes several things about the pattern. Onset has ranged from a few days to as long as a year after starting. Most reported cases have been mild to moderate, with rapid recovery once the drug is stopped. Some have been severe and potentially life-threatening [SRC-0017].

Two observations from that source deserve particular attention, because they describe a problem that no amount of individual caution can solve alone.

The first is that people taking fenbendazole often do so without telling their oncologist, and may be reluctant to mention it. The second is that liver injury is not unusual during cancer treatment, so when it appears, it is likely to be attributed to chemotherapy, to immunotherapy, or to the cancer itself [SRC-0017]. The 2026 case report cited above exists precisely because distinguishing fenbendazole-associated liver injury from immunotherapy-related hepatitis required a formal, structured causality assessment [SRC-0023].

Follow that through. An undisclosed compound causes liver injury. The injury is attributed to the cancer treatment. The cancer treatment is paused, reduced, or stopped, and the patient may be given immune-suppressing drugs they did not need. The harm in that sequence is not only the liver injury. It is the disruption of treatment that was working.

WHY THE PROTOCOLS VARY

Anyone who spends an hour reading about this will notice something odd. There is no single protocol. There are many, and they differ from one another in nearly every respect: how much, how often, for how long, with what taken alongside, and with what breaks in between.

This book will not describe any of them, and the reason is not squeamishness. It is that describing a regimen implies that someone knows what the right regimen is, and no one does.

Consider what a dose actually represents in medicine. It is the output of pharmacokinetic studies establishing what the body does with a compound, dose-finding studies establishing what can be tolerated, and trials establishing what quantity produces the intended effect. For fenbendazole in humans with cancer, none of that work exists. So where do the numbers in circulating protocols come from? They are derived from animal labelling, from one man's personal practice, and from subsequent adaptation by people who had no more information than anyone else.

The variation is therefore not a menu of options. It is a visible symptom of an absent evidence base. In a field with real data, protocols converge, because they are all being pulled toward the same measured answer. Where they diverge freely, it is usually because there is nothing to converge on.

There is a second thing the variation reveals. Protocols have accumulated components over time, gaining supplements and additional compounds as the online conversation has evolved. Each addition makes the attribution problem worse. If someone takes a compound alongside conventional treatment and several supplements, and does well, the number of possible explanations has grown, not shrunk. The protocols have become less interpretable as they have become more elaborate.

Underneath the question of how much lies a question about what, and it receives even less attention. Chapter 1 introduced formulation as one of the details that has to be pinned down before a claim means anything. Here it is unusually consequential.

Products made for animals are manufactured to veterinary standards. Those standards are real and they are enforced. But they were written for a different purpose. The goal is to deliver a reliable dose to a species that is not human, often in a form meant to be mixed into feed or given as a paste. The testing, the inactive ingredients, the labelling requirements, and the tolerances are all set with that use in mind. None of it was designed around a person taking the product daily for months.

Beyond the regulated products there is a further layer. Where demand exists, sellers appear, and material sold online may not have come through any regulated veterinary supply chain at all. For a person taking something over a long period, the question of whether each unit contains what it claims, and only what it claims, is not a pedantic one.

The practical consequence is that even the accounts people find persuasive are difficult to interpret. If two people follow what they believe is the same protocol using different products from different sources, they may not have taken the same thing. That uncertainty sits underneath every anecdote in this area, and it is one more reason the compiled testimonials cannot be assembled into evidence.

THE SAFETY QUESTIONS NOBODY HAS ANSWERED

It is common to read that fenbendazole is safe because it has been given to animals for decades with few problems. That statement is true and largely irrelevant, and it is worth being precise about why.

Safety established in animals is safety in those animals, at those exposures, for those durations, for that purpose. A dog treated for worms receives the drug for a short course, in a body that is not fighting cancer, and is not simultaneously receiving chemotherapy, immunotherapy, or eight other prescriptions. Every one of those differences changes the question.

It helps to look at what the animal safety record actually consists of. One of the studies frequently invoked examined twenty-eight cats given fenbendazole for nine days at up to five times the recommended dose and three times the recommended duration. No adverse events were observed and the blood tests remained unchanged throughout [SRC-0017]. That is a reassuring result and it was properly conducted.

Now notice what it establishes. Twenty-eight animals. Nine days. Cats. Healthy cats, not cats undergoing cancer treatment. It is a good study of exactly the question it asked, and it says nothing whatever about a human being taking the compound continuously for a year alongside immunotherapy. When someone writes that fenbendazole has an excellent safety record, this is the sort of evidence underneath the sentence, and it is worth knowing that before deciding how much weight the sentence can hold.

There is a related point about how safety information accumulates. For an approved human medicine, uncommon harms are detected because large numbers of people are treated under supervision, adverse events are recorded, and there is a system for reporting them. For a compound taken privately, outside medical care, and often undisclosed, no such system operates. Harms are only detected when someone becomes ill enough to reach a hospital and a clinician thinks to ask the right question. That means the published cases described in this chapter are, almost by definition, the visible portion of something whose full size is unknown. It would be wrong to claim that the true figure is high. It would be equally wrong to read the small number of published reports as a reassuring measurement, because nobody is counting.

Here is what is not known, stated plainly.

What happens to fenbendazole in a human body over months of continuous use has not been characterised. Whether the concentrations reached in a person are anywhere near those at which laboratory activity was observed is unknown. What it does when combined with specific cancer treatments has not been studied. Whether it interferes with the effectiveness of those treatments, in either direction, has not been established. What happens with prolonged use in an older adult with reduced liver or kidney function, taking several other medicines, has not been studied at all.

What is known is the liver signal, and it is not theoretical. It comes from published cases in real patients, it has been assessed by a national resource as a probable cause of clinically apparent injury, and in some cases it has been severe [SRC-0017].

Notice the asymmetry that has emerged. The claims of benefit rest on cells, animals, and individual accounts. The evidence of harm rests on documented human cases. That does not mean the compound cannot help anyone. It means the two sides of the ledger are not made of the same material, and any honest summary has to say so.

WHAT WOULD HAVE TO CHANGE

It would be easy to end this chapter with a shrug. That would be inaccurate, because the question of what would resolve this is entirely answerable.

Human pharmacokinetic data would be the first requirement: a proper study establishing what happens to fenbendazole in the body of a person with cancer, and whether a meaningful concentration reaches a tumour. Without that, everything else is speculation.

A dose-finding safety study would follow, establishing what can be tolerated and for how long, in patients rather than in healthy volunteers.

Then a study designed to detect a signal in a defined group of patients, with a stated endpoint and a predefined benchmark. Then, if the signal appeared, a comparative trial against standard treatment.

Along the way, one specific question would need its own answer: whether fenbendazole interferes with the cancer treatments patients are actually receiving. Given that most people taking it are taking it alongside something else, this may be the most practically urgent question of all, and it is currently unaddressed.

None of that is impossible, and none of it requires anyone's permission from a conspiracy. It requires funding, patients willing to enrol, and researchers willing to run it. If those studies are done and they show benefit, this chapter will be wrong, and that will be a good day. The point of setting out the requirements is that it makes the current position falsifiable, which is more than can be said for the claim that the evidence is being hidden.

That claim deserves a fair hearing rather than a dismissal, because a real observation sits underneath it.

Clinical trials are expensive. They are usually funded by whoever stands to sell the resulting product, and a compound with no patent protection offers no one that prospect. This produces a genuine structural gap: there are compounds that might be worth testing and that no commercial sponsor has any reason to test. Researchers in the drug repurposing field say this openly, and it is one of the main arguments they make when seeking public and charitable funding. So the frustration is not paranoid. It is pointing at something true about how research gets paid for.

Where the argument goes wrong is in the leap from *nobody has a financial incentive to fund this* to *the answer is being concealed*. Those are very different claims. The first is an observation about economics and is largely correct. The second requires that someone knows the answer, and nothing in this chapter suggests anyone does.

There are also non-commercial routes, and they are not hypothetical. Government agencies, cancer charities, academic centres, and dedicated repurposing organisations fund trials of off-patent compounds. Those routes are slower and more competitive than industry funding, and they involve proposals being judged against other proposals. A compound can fail to attract that funding for unglamorous reasons: thin human pharmacokinetic data, an unclear formulation, uncertainty about what dose to even test.

It is also worth noticing what a major oncology society actually said in 2026. It did not say the question was closed or unworthy. It said the evidence does not currently support use outside a trial, and that well-designed comparative trials would be needed to establish whether there is any benefit worth having [SRC-0026]. That is a call for the research, published by the professional body that would have to conduct it. It is difficult to reconcile with the idea that the field is refusing to look.

Where This Leaves Us

Claim commonly made	What the evidence actually supports	What remains unknown or unstudied
Fenbendazole cures cancer	Nothing in the published literature supports this	Whether it has any effect on any cancer in humans
Studies prove it kills cancer cells	Cell and animal studies report activity in some models	Whether relevant concentrations are reachable in a person
Animal studies show it shrinks tumours	One study reported inhibition; another found none; a third found an effect only combined with vitamins	Which result, if any, predicts a human response
A man was cured by it	One documented remission in a man simultaneously receiving immunotherapy	What each intervention contributed
Published case reports confirm it	A small number exist; the most prominent was retracted in January 2026	Whether the reported responses were caused by the compound

Claim commonly made	What the evidence actually supports	What remains unknown or unstudied
It is safe because animals take it	Well tolerated in animals, short-term, for deworming	Safety in humans, long-term, during cancer treatment
It has no side effects in people	Published human cases describe liver injury, some severe	How often injury occurs, and who is most at risk
Doctors will not study it because it is cheap	Reviews and a major oncology society have publicly called for trials	Why the trials have not yet been funded and run

The verdict, stated as precisely as the evidence allows:

Fenbendazole is a veterinary antiparasitic. It has documented laboratory activity against cancer cells in some models. In animals, the results have been inconsistent, with one study reporting tumour inhibition, one finding none, and one finding an effect only in combination with something else. Its behaviour in the human body has never been properly characterised. No clinical trial of it as a cancer treatment has been completed in people. A small number of individual case reports describe tumour response, and the most prominent of those was retracted in January 2026. Meanwhile a growing and consistent set of published human cases describes drug-induced liver injury, some of it severe.

Put more simply: it has not been shown to treat cancer in people, and it has not been shown to be safe in people taking it for months alongside cancer treatment. Both statements are about the absence of studies rather than the presence of disproof. Neither should be inflated into something stronger than it is.

Read that verdict carefully, because it will be quoted back at you in two distorted forms.

It does not say that fenbendazole is worthless, that the researchers who studied it wasted their time, or that anyone taking it has been fooled. The laboratory findings are real, the mechanistic reasoning is coherent, and the people asking these questions are not being foolish.

It also does not say that the evidence is merely incomplete and that hope is therefore reasonable in the meantime. The evidence for benefit in humans is not thin; on the central question it is absent. And the evidence of harm, while limited in quantity, is of a stronger kind than anything on the other side of the ledger, because it consists of documented human cases rather than cells and mice.

Holding both of those at once is uncomfortable, and it is the accurate position. Uncertainty here is not symmetrical, and treating it as though the two possibilities were evenly balanced would misrepresent what has actually been found.

SIX QUESTIONS WORTH ASKING

If you are considering this, or if someone you care about already is, these are questions worth raising with the oncology team. They are designed to produce information rather than to win an argument.

1. Is there anything in my current treatment that fenbendazole could interact with, either through the liver enzymes it shares, or by adding to the same side effects?

2. If I were taking it and developed a problem, how would you tell whether it came from the fenbendazole or from my cancer treatment?

3. Is there anything in my medical history, particularly my liver function, that would make this riskier for me specifically than for someone else?

4. Are there any trials, of this compound or of anything in the same class, that I would be eligible for?

5. If I decide to take it anyway, what would you want to know, and how often would you want to hear from me?

6. What would change your mind about this, and what evidence would you want to see?

That fifth question is worth emphasising. The choice is not between telling your oncologist and taking it. Concealment does not make it safer; it removes the only person who could recognise a problem early and prevent your actual treatment from being interrupted for the wrong reason.

Some people hesitate at this because they expect to be judged, or lectured, or told to stop. That fear is not unfounded, and the conversation is not always handled well. But the published cases in this chapter show what the alternative costs. In each of them, the injury was recognised because somebody eventually asked the right question and got a truthful answer. In at least one, working out where the problem came from required a formal investigation that would have been unnecessary had the information been available from the start.

You are allowed to disagree with your oncologist. You are allowed to decide something they would not have chosen. What is hard to defend is leaving them to work in the dark, because the person that mostly disadvantages is you.

WHERE THIS LEADS

Fenbendazole has never been given to a person in a clinical trial for cancer.

That single fact makes it the simplest of the three compounds to assess, because the evidence base is nearly empty. The other two are harder, and in an instructive way. Ivermectin and mebendazole are approved human medicines, both have been studied in people, and both have generated human data in cancer settings.

That makes them a more complicated story than fenbendazole, not a clearer one. It also creates the trap that this book has been building toward: when evidence about one compound is used to make a case about another.

That is where the next chapter begins.

CHAPTER 3
IVERMECTIN AND MEBENDAZOLE: A MORE COMPLICATED PICTURE

WHY THESE TWO GET GROUPED WITH THE FIRST

Fenbendazole was, in one sense, easy. The evidence base for it in humans is nearly empty, so the appraisal was mostly a matter of describing an absence.

Ivermectin and mebendazole are harder, and the difficulty runs in an unexpected direction.

Both are approved human medicines. Both have decades of safety data in people. Both have been given to cancer patients inside real clinical trials, with consent forms, defined endpoints, and published results. There is more genuine human evidence here than for fenbendazole by a wide margin.

That extra evidence is exactly what makes this chapter more difficult rather than less. When there is nothing to examine, the honest answer is short. When there is something, you have to read it properly, and reading it properly means noticing what each study was built to find out and what it actually found.

There is also a trap waiting here, and it is the reason this chapter exists at all. Because these three compounds are discussed together online, evidence about one is constantly used to make a case about another. A human trial of mebendazole becomes support for fenbendazole. A laboratory paper on ivermectin becomes support for all three. Chapter 1 named this problem. This chapter is where you will see it in operation.

One more thing before starting. These two compounds are not the same as each other either. Mebendazole is a benzimidazole and is chemically related to fenbendazole. Ivermectin is not a benzimidazole at all. It belongs to a completely different chemical family, works through a different mechanism against parasites, and has a different safety profile. Grouping the three together is a habit of the internet, not a fact about pharmacology.

It is worth naming what actually holds the group together, because it is not chemistry. It is a story.

The story is that these are old, cheap, off-patent antiparasitic drugs that nobody has a financial reason to investigate, and that this is why you have not heard about them from your doctor. Chapter 2 examined that argument and found a real observation inside it. Trials are expensive, off-patent compounds attract no commercial sponsor, and there is a genuine structural gap in what gets studied.

But notice what the story does once it takes hold. It creates a category defined by a grievance rather than by pharmacology. Anything that fits the shape of the grievance joins the category, and evidence about any member starts to feel like evidence about the category itself. That is how a mouse study of one compound becomes reassurance about a different one.

This chapter takes each compound on its own terms, which means the group has to be taken apart first.

IVERMECTIN: WHAT IT IS AND WHY THE INTEREST AROSE

Ivermectin is a genuine success story in medicine, and that is worth saying plainly before anything else.

It belongs to a group of compounds called avermectins, discovered in the 1970s and approved for human use in the United States in the 1980s. It has been given to many millions of people, mostly in large public health programmes against parasitic diseases. Its discovery was recognised with a Nobel Prize in 2015. Its human safety record at approved doses is, by any standard, excellent.

In the United States it is approved in tablet form for two parasitic infections: intestinal strongyloidiasis and onchocerciasis, also called river blindness. Topical formulations are approved separately for other conditions. It is not approved to treat any cancer.

The scientific interest in ivermectin and cancer is real and it predates the pandemic. Laboratory researchers reported that it appeared to act on several different cellular systems at once. The list is long and includes mitochondrial function, a protein pump that cancer cells use to expel drugs, several signalling pathways involved in growth, and the population of cells sometimes called cancer stem cells. Reviews of this literature describe inhibition of cell growth and induction of cell death across many cancer types in laboratory models [SRC-0029].

That breadth is part of the appeal, and it is also the first thing worth questioning. A compound that appears to affect a great many different systems may be exquisitely versatile. It may also be doing something non-specific. Chapter 1 warned that a mechanistic explanation can feel more like proof than it is. A long list of mechanisms can feel like a very long proof, and it is not one.

There is one more thing to say about ivermectin, and skipping it would be dishonest.

For several years this compound was at the centre of an enormous public argument about a different disease. That argument was bitter, it became political, and it left almost everyone with strong feelings about the word itself. Many people concluded that ivermectin had been unfairly dismissed. Many others concluded that any interest in it was a warning sign about the person expressing it.

Both of those reflexes will get in the way here, and both should be set down.

The cancer question is a separate question. It has its own laboratory literature, which is older than the pandemic. It has its own trials, with their own designs and endpoints. Whatever you concluded about the antiviral argument tells you nothing about whether this compound affects a tumour, and importing that conclusion in either direction is exactly the kind of shortcut this book is trying to replace.

What the earlier episode did leave behind is useful, though. It generated a great deal of careful work on one specific question: what concentrations of ivermectin a human body can actually reach. That question turns out to be the centre of the cancer story too.

THE CONCENTRATION QUESTION

Here is where the ivermectin story becomes genuinely interesting, and where most coverage of it goes quiet.

Recall from Chapter 1 that a laboratory result comes attached to a concentration. The compound was present around the cells at a certain amount. The question that decides everything is whether a human body can reach and hold that amount.

For ivermectin, this question has been asked directly and it has not been settled.

Some researchers have argued that the answer is yes. One study set out to test this directly. It asked whether ivermectin's antitumour effects appear at concentrations a person could actually achieve. The researchers examined a large panel of cancer cell lines at a fixed concentration. Several were sensitive, particularly certain breast and ovarian lines. The authors concluded that the effects were observable at clinically feasible concentrations and that this supported developing ivermectin as a repositioned cancer drug [SRC-0030]. Review articles have made the same argument, describing the typical laboratory concentration as attainable based on human pharmacokinetic data [SRC-0029].

Other researchers disagree, and their disagreement is not casual. The same question was fought over at length during the pandemic, when ivermectin was proposed as an antiviral. Analyses at the time reached a different conclusion. The concentrations producing antiviral activity in a dish were far above anything reachable with approved oral dosing in people. Laboratory work published later suggested that some of the in-vitro activity might reflect a non-specific effect on cell membranes at high concentrations rather than a targeted action.

You do not need to resolve this dispute to use it. What matters is that it exists, that it is a dispute among researchers rather than between researchers and the public, and that it sits directly underneath every claim built on ivermectin's laboratory data. When someone tells you that studies show ivermectin kills cancer cells, the unasked question is: at what concentration, and can a person get there?

Notice also what this dispute does not settle. It does not show that ivermectin is useless. It shows that the most important preclinical question about it is contested. That is a reason for a trial, which is precisely what happened next.

One further caution belongs to this literature. Among the preclinical papers frequently cited in support of ivermectin is at least one that has since been retracted. That does not taint the rest of the field, and retractions occur across all of biomedical research. But it is a reminder that the reference list under a confident online claim is not self-verifying, and that a paper's status can change after the video citing it was made.

There is also a general point about breadth worth stating plainly. When a compound is reported to act on mitochondria, drug efflux pumps, several growth pathways, and stem cell populations, one possible explanation is that it is a remarkably versatile agent. Another is that at high concentrations it disturbs cell membranes and therefore appears to disrupt whatever anyone happens to measure. Researchers have raised exactly this possibility. It does not mean the findings are worthless. It means that the number of reported mechanisms is not, by itself, evidence of anything, and a reader counting them is not measuring strength.

WHAT HUMAN TRIALS OF IVERMECTIN HAVE FOUND

Ivermectin has been given to cancer patients inside a registered clinical trial. This is the single biggest difference between it and fenbendazole, and it deserves to be reported accurately rather than triumphantly.

The trial is a phase I/II study combining ivermectin with an immune checkpoint inhibitor in patients with metastatic triple-negative breast cancer who had already progressed on previous treatment. Preliminary results from the first patients enrolled were presented at a major oncology meeting in 2025 [SRC-0031].

Here is what was reported. Nine patients had been enrolled and eight were evaluable for response. Of those eight, one had a partial response, one had stable disease, and six had progressive disease. The median time before the cancer progressed was about two and a half months. A measure called the four-month clinical benefit rate came out at just under forty percent, and the confidence interval around that figure was extremely wide. Side effects were mostly mild. The authors concluded that the combination was safe and well tolerated, that the clinical benefit rate was encouraging in this heavily pretreated group, and that continued investigation was warranted [SRC-0031].

Now read that carefully, because it is a good exercise.

The study was a dose-escalation study. Its primary job was to establish safety and dosing, not to determine whether the combination helps. It had no comparison group, so there is no way to know what would have happened to these patients on the immunotherapy alone. Everyone was receiving a checkpoint inhibitor as well as ivermectin, which is the co-intervention problem again. And with eight evaluable patients, the confidence interval around any response figure is so wide as to be almost uninformative. Chapter 1 explained why sample size governs what a study can detect. This is what that looks like in practice.

Notice too that six of eight patients progressed. That is not a scandal and it is not hidden; it is in the published abstract. It is simply what happens when you read the whole result instead of the conclusion sentence.

Two terms in that report deserve unpacking, because both are routinely over-read.

A **dose-escalation study** gives the first small group of participants a low dose. If that is tolerated, the next group receives more, and so on, until either the target dose is reached or unacceptable side effects appear. The purpose is to find out what people can take. Response measurements are collected along the way and are genuinely useful, but they are a by-product. Some participants in such a study, by design, receive doses that nobody expects to do anything.

A **clinical benefit rate** counts the proportion of patients whose disease responded *or* stayed stable for some period. It is a legitimate and widely used measure. It is also softer than it sounds, because stable disease is doing a great deal of the work. A cancer that has not grown over a few months may reflect a treatment effect. It may also reflect a cancer that was growing slowly. Without a comparison group, the two cannot be told apart.

So when a headline says that a substantial share of patients experienced clinical benefit, the honest translation is narrower: that share had disease which had not clearly worsened by the time it was measured. That is worth knowing. It is not the same as improvement, and it is a long way from survival.

The authors' own language was measured. They said the combination was tolerable and that investigation should continue. They did not say it worked. When this trial is described online, the word *encouraging* frequently arrives without the eight patients attached to it.

A larger randomised study of ivermectin with checkpoint inhibitors in solid tumours has been planned, with an estimated start in mid-2026 and a target of around eighty patients [SRC-0032]. As Chapter 1 explained, a registry entry means a question is being asked. It is not an answer, and at the time of writing there is no result to report.

The professional position, as of a clinical notice issued in May 2026, is that no robust peer-reviewed clinical evidence demonstrates that ivermectin is safe or effective for treating any human cancer, and that comparative trials would be needed to establish whether it has any benefit worth the harms [SRC-0026].

MEBENDAZOLE: WHAT IT IS AND WHY THE INTEREST AROSE

Mebendazole is the compound most likely to surprise you, in both directions.

It is an approved human medicine, and has been in the United States since 1974. It is used for common intestinal worm infections, and at those doses and durations it is very well tolerated. It is a benzimidazole, which makes it a chemical relative of fenbendazole, and it works against parasites in the same way, by binding tubulin.

There is a detail about mebendazole in the United States that cuts against the story holding these three compounds together, and it is worth knowing. Although mebendazole is an old, long-approved, off-patent medicine, the original US product was discontinued years ago. For some time there has been a single approved mebendazole product on the American market, with no approved generic version. Sole-source products with low prescription volumes are frequently expensive, and this one is no exception. Availability has also been inconsistent, since pharmacies have little reason to stock a costly item that rarely moves.

So the picture of a cheap drug sitting on every pharmacy shelf, ignored only because nobody can profit from it, does not describe mebendazole in the United States. That does not make the wider concern about off-patent research funding wrong. It is a reminder that the story travels ahead of the facts, and that the facts vary by compound and by country.

The interest in mebendazole and cancer is the oldest and most academically established of the three. Research groups at major universities have worked on it for over a decade. Much of that work has focused on brain tumours, for a specific and sensible reason: laboratory studies indicated that mebendazole can cross into brain tissue at concentrations that might matter, which is a serious obstacle for most drugs and a genuine point in its favour.

Preclinical work reported that mebendazole extended survival in animal models of glioblastoma and other brain cancers. Studies also reported activity in colorectal cancer models. Others reported interference with the formation of new blood vessels that tumours use to feed themselves. Several separate research groups, working independently, reported findings in the same direction.

This is a stronger and more coherent preclinical case than exists for either of the other two compounds. It came from academic laboratories, it was reproduced across groups, and it was specific enough to point toward a particular disease. It is exactly the sort of preclinical work that ought to lead to human trials.

The brain-penetration point deserves emphasis, because it is not a minor technical detail. The brain is protected by a barrier that keeps most substances in the bloodstream out of it. That barrier is one of the main reasons brain tumours are so difficult to treat: a drug can be highly effective against tumour cells in a dish and completely useless in a patient because it never arrives. A compound reported to cross into brain tissue at meaningful concentrations has cleared an obstacle that stops many candidates.

There is a wrinkle here that illustrates the formulation problem from

Chapter 1, and it is unusually concrete. Mebendazole can exist in different crystalline forms. Those forms are absorbed very differently. Laboratory work found they were not equivalent in reaching brain tumours in animals. In other words, two products containing the same named compound may not deliver the same thing. This is a difference between manufactured versions of an approved human medicine, established by researchers who needed to know which version to test. It is worth holding onto the next time someone describes two products as the same drug.

So the preclinical case was strong, coherent, reproduced, and specific. It pointed clearly toward a human trial. And it got one. That is why mebendazole is the most instructive of the three.

WHAT HUMAN TRIALS OF MEBENDAZOLE HAVE FOUND

Two published trials matter here. They point in different directions, and the second one matters more.

The phase 1 study. A single-centre dose-escalation study enrolled twenty-four patients with newly diagnosed high-grade brain tumours. Mebendazole was added to standard treatment, not substituted for it. The study escalated through several dose levels, with most patients treated at the highest level studied [SRC-0033].

The safety findings were the point of the study, and they were informative. Four patients at the highest dose developed significant elevations in liver enzymes after about a month. These reversed when the dose was lowered or the drug stopped. Plasma levels of the drug varied considerably between patients. The authors concluded that mebendazole at the doses studied showed long-term safety and acceptable toxicity, and that further studies were needed to determine whether it actually helps [SRC-0033].

The study also reported survival figures, and this is where care is required. Median overall survival was about twenty-one months, with a substantial fraction of patients alive at two years. Those numbers look encouraging. But this was a single-arm study with no comparison group, so there is nothing to compare them against except historical figures from other populations, which is not a reliable comparison.

The paper also reported that patients who took mebendazole for more than a month had longer progression-free survival than those who took it for less than a month. This comparison is worth pausing on, because it is the kind of thing that travels well online and means less than it appears to. Patients who stayed on a drug longer are, on average, patients who were doing better. Those who came off early often did so because they deteriorated or could not tolerate it. The comparison is therefore partly measuring who was well enough to continue. It cannot be read as an effect of the drug.

The authors themselves were careful. They noted that mebendazole has not been optimised for oncology, that efficacy has not been established in a randomised trial, that the side effects include liver enzyme elevations and low blood counts which require detection and dose adjustment, and that the bioavailability of different mebendazole preparations varies substantially, making some formulations likely unsuitable for oncology patients [SRC-0033]. That last point is the formulation issue from Chapter 1, raised by trial investigators about an approved human drug.

The randomised trial. This is the most important piece of human evidence in this entire book, and it is very rarely mentioned in the material that brought most readers here.

A team in India ran a randomised open-label phase II trial in patients with recurrent glioblastoma. Eighty-eight patients were randomised, forty-four to each arm. Both arms received mebendazole; the arms differed in which standard chemotherapy it was combined with. The primary endpoint was overall survival at nine months, and the researchers had committed in advance to a benchmark. A nine-month survival of fifty-five percent or more in either arm would justify further investigation. A figure below thirty-five percent would mean it was not worth pursuing [SRC-0034].

The result: neither arm reached the benchmark. Nine-month overall survival was about thirty-seven percent in one arm and forty-five percent in the other. The authors' interpretation was direct. The addition of mebendazole failed to achieve the pre-set benchmark. They noted that this was probably influenced by a substantial proportion of patients entering the trial in poor general condition [SRC-0034].

Everything Chapter 1 taught applies here at once. There was a predefined benchmark, committed to before the data came in. There was randomisation. The result was published whether or not it was welcome. And the result did not meet the mark.

Read it precisely, though. This trial does not prove mebendazole does nothing. It was a phase II trial in one very difficult cancer, in patients many of whom were already frail, with no arm that omitted mebendazole entirely. A different cancer, an earlier stage, or a different design might produce a different answer. The authors did not claim otherwise.

But it is real evidence, and it counts. Chapter 1 was explicit that unfavourable results deserve the same reading as favourable ones. Here is the compound with the strongest preclinical case, the most academic backing, and demonstrated ability to reach the target tissue. It was tested properly, against a benchmark set in advance, and it did not clear it.

That result is almost entirely absent from online discussion of these compounds. Ask yourself why.

Other human work on mebendazole exists and points the same way: interesting enough to continue, not yet showing benefit. Further early-phase studies have been conducted, including in children with brain tumours that had returned after treatment, and in adults with recurrent high-grade glioma. There are also individual case reports, including one long-cited account of prolonged disease control in a rare adrenal cancer.

Chapter 1's framework applies to all of it in the same way. Early-phase studies establish tolerability and dosing. Case reports describe individuals and cannot establish cause. None of this is nothing, and none of it is evidence of benefit. It is the ordinary, unglamorous middle of a research programme that has been running for more than a decade without yet producing a positive comparative result.

THE COHORT STUDY EVERYONE IS CITING

In 2026 a study appeared that changed the shape of these conversations, and it requires careful handling.

The paper reported outcomes in a group of cancer patients taking ivermectin and mebendazole together. It was published in an indexed, peer-reviewed oncology journal in May 2026. It was announced as the largest human study of these compounds ever conducted, and its headline figure spread rapidly: more than eighty percent of participants reported that their cancer had disappeared, regressed, or stabilised [SRC-0035].

If you have encountered any claim about these drugs in the past few months, there is a good chance it traced back to this paper. So let us do the work.

What the study was. Just under two hundred cancer patients were prescribed a combination of ivermectin and mebendazole off-label, through a telemedicine platform, by licensed providers. Data were collected by voluntary digital surveys at the start and again at about six months. Of the initial group, roughly sixty-two percent completed the follow-up survey. The outcomes reported were self-reported cancer status, adherence, and side effects [SRC-0035].

What the headline number is made of. Before examining the design, look at how the figure itself was built. The widely quoted percentage combines three different outcomes into one total: patients reporting no evidence of disease, patients reporting that their tumour had shrunk, and patients reporting that their cancer had stayed the same.

That third category is doing an enormous amount of work. As explained above, stable disease over six months can reflect a treatment effect, or a slowly growing cancer, or a cancer already controlled by conventional treatment the person was also receiving. Combining it with remission under a single heading produces a large, impressive number that describes a mixture of very different situations.

This is not a hidden manoeuvre; the composition is stated in the paper. But when the figure travels, the composition does not travel with it. What most readers hear is that four in five people got better, and that is not what was measured.

What that design can establish. Now apply the ladder. This is an observational study with no comparison group, and its outcomes are patient-reported rather than confirmed by imaging or pathology. It can describe what a group of people said happened to them. It cannot establish that the compounds caused any of it.

Four specific problems compound that.

There was no control group, so there is no way to know what would have happened to these patients otherwise. Nearly all of them were presumably also receiving conventional cancer treatment, which is the attribution problem in a large form.

The outcomes were self-reported. "My cancer regressed" is a statement about what a person believes and has been told, filtered through hope and through what they understood at their last appointment. It is not a measurement.

Nearly four in ten participants did not complete the follow-up survey. Chapter 1's point about selection applies with unusual force here. People who are doing well are more likely to fill in a survey about a treatment they chose than people who have deteriorated or died. Whatever the true picture, the responding group is not a random sample of the starting group.

And the patients were recruited through a commercial platform that prescribes and supplies the combination. That is a financial relationship between the source of the data and the product being evaluated.

What happened next. In June 2026, the journal's editorial board issued a formal Expression of Concern about the paper [SRC-0036].

Chapter 1 defined that notice. It alerts readers to credible concerns about a paper's reliability that fall short of retraction, or where conclusive evidence cannot be obtained quickly. The paper has not been withdrawn. It has also not been cleared.

The notice states its reasons. After publication, serious concerns were raised by the international medical community about the verifiability and statistical reliability of the underlying dataset, and about its ethical oversight. The authors responded in correspondence, clarifying that the cohort was not drawn from an unverified consumer survey but consisted of provider-screened patients enrolled through a structured clinical workflow [SRC-0036].

The editorial board's reasoning is worth understanding, because it is a clear statement of a principle this whole book has been building toward. The board acknowledged that the authors had been transparent about the limits of self-reported data. It then said that transparency was not sufficient. A study published in a peer-reviewed oncology journal that reports a specific benefit rate and specific percentages of tumour regression must rest on a verifiably real clinical foundation and must meet established ethical frameworks for research involving human subjects. Disclosing limitations does not exempt a dataset from the requirements of verifiability and independent ethical oversight [SRC-0036].

The journal has opened a formal audit. It will examine the ethics-committee approval or exemption documentation, source-verified clinical records confirming the baseline cancer diagnoses of the participants, and objective medical documentation supporting the reported tumour regressions. The Expression of Concern will remain attached to the paper, in the journal and in the indexing databases, while that audit proceeds. The board also stated that it does not endorse the unvalidated off-label use of medications for unapproved cancer indications [SRC-0036].

How to hold this. Be precise, because both distortions are already circulating.

This is not proof that the study was fraudulent. No such finding has been made, the audit is not complete, and the authors have offered an explanation which the journal is examining.

It is also not a technicality, and it is not evidence of persecution. The concerns are about whether the underlying data can be verified and whether the study met the ethical requirements for research on human subjects. Those are foundational questions, not procedural ones.

What follows practically is straightforward. A paper carrying an Expression of Concern cannot be used as though it were settled evidence. It sits in a suspended state, and treating it as established misrepresents where it stands. If the audit clears it, that will be worth knowing. If it does not, that will be worth knowing too.

There is a lesson here beyond this one paper. The headline figure travelled around the world within days. The Expression of Concern, issued a few weeks later, travelled almost nowhere. If you had saved the citation and checked it, you would have found the notice in under a minute. This is exactly the check Chapter 1 asked you to make, and this is exactly why.

It is also worth asking what would make a study like this convincing, because the answer is not out of reach.

Participants' diagnoses would need to be confirmed from medical records rather than taken from a form. Outcomes would need to come from imaging and pathology read by someone who did not know what the patient was taking, rather than from what the patient wrote in a survey. Conventional treatment would need to be recorded in detail, so that its contribution could at least be described. Everyone who started would need to be accounted for at the end, including those who died or withdrew. Ethical approval would need to be documented before enrolment rather than explained afterwards. And ideally there would be a comparison group.

None of that is exotic. It is ordinary clinical research, and it is done routinely by academic centres and cooperative groups. The gap between what this study did and what would have made it convincing is not a matter of funding or of access to patients. It is a matter of design.

That is a genuinely frustrating conclusion, because a well-designed version of this study would be enormously valuable. Thousands of people are already taking these compounds. Following them properly, with confirmed diagnoses and objective outcomes, would produce real information about a question a lot of people want answered. The opportunity is there. It has not yet been taken.

WHAT "APPROVED AND SAFE" DOES AND DOES NOT BUY YOU

There is one argument for ivermectin and mebendazole that sounds decisive and is not. It goes like this: unlike fenbendazole, these are approved human medicines with excellent safety records, so the risk of trying them is minimal.

The first half of that is true. The second half does not follow, and understanding why matters more than anything else in this chapter.

A safety record is a record of specific exposures. Ivermectin's outstanding record comes from many millions of doses given for parasitic infections. Those are usually single doses, or a very short course, in people who are otherwise well. Mebendazole's record comes from short courses for intestinal worms. In both cases, what has been established is that a particular amount, given for a particular length of time, to broadly healthy people, is very well tolerated.

Now change each of those variables. Cancer protocols involve larger amounts, taken for months rather than days, by people whose bodies are under considerable strain, alongside treatments that place their own demands on the liver and the bone marrow. The safety record does not extend to that situation, because that situation has not been studied at the same scale.

This is not speculation. When mebendazole was given at oncology doses in a clinical trial, several patients developed significant liver enzyme elevations after about a month, and dose reductions or discontinuation were required. Those patients were being monitored, in a trial, with investigators watching for exactly that. The signal appeared anyway. The same trial's authors specifically noted low blood counts as a concern requiring detection and dose adjustment.

So the accurate statement is narrower than the reassuring one. These compounds are very safe when used as approved. What happens at oncology exposures, for months, in a person receiving cancer treatment, is a different question, and the evidence available on it comes mostly from trials in which people were being watched carefully. That is not the situation of someone taking them privately.

There is a specific asymmetry worth naming, too. Fenbendazole's risks are visible in published case reports precisely because it is not approved and its use is invisible to any monitoring system, so harm only surfaces when someone becomes ill enough to be written up. For approved drugs used off-label outside medical care, the same blind spot exists. Approval does not create surveillance of uses that nobody reports.

THREE COMPOUNDS, SIDE BY SIDE

	Fenbendazole	Ivermectin	Mebendazole
Approval status	Veterinary only; no human approval	Approved human drug, for two parasitic infections	Approved human drug, for intestinal worms
Human safety data	None from formal study; published cases of liver injury	Extensive at approved doses; limited at oncology exposures	Extensive at antiparasitic doses; trial data show liver enzyme elevations at higher doses
Preclinical evidence	Mixed: one positive, one negative, one only in combination	Broad activity reported; whether concentrations are achievable is disputed	Strongest and most reproduced; brain penetration reported
Human cancer trials	None completed	One early-phase trial reported; a randomised trial planned	Phase 1 completed; a randomised phase II did not meet its benchmark
Approved for cancer	No	No	No

Read the bottom row first. It is the only row that is identical across all three.

Now read the fourth row, because it contains the finding this chapter exists to deliver. The compound with the most human evidence is the one where a properly designed trial returned a negative result. More evidence did not mean more support. It meant a clearer answer, and the answer was not the hoped-for one.

WHY EVIDENCE CANNOT BE PASSED BETWEEN THEM

You now have enough detail to see why the transfer of evidence between these compounds is not a small error.

Consider what would have to be true for a mebendazole result to tell you something about fenbendazole. The two would need to behave similarly in the human body, reaching similar concentrations in similar tissues. Nothing establishes that. Mebendazole's absorption and distribution in humans have been studied, including in cancer patients. Fenbendazole's have not been characterised at all. The one thing we know about fenbendazole's behaviour, that it is poorly absorbed by design, is a reason to expect a difference rather than a similarity.

Now consider ivermectin. It is not a benzimidazole. It does not share the tubulin-binding mechanism that connects the other two. Its proposed anti-cancer mechanisms are a different list entirely. Using an ivermectin finding to support a claim about fenbendazole is not a stretch of the evidence; it is a category error.

There is a further asymmetry that matters. Mebendazole is the only one of the three that has been through a randomised trial against a predefined benchmark, and that trial was negative. If evidence really did transfer between these compounds, that negative result would transfer too. In practice, the transfer is only ever performed in one direction. Favourable findings migrate freely from one compound to another. Unfavourable findings stay put.

That one-way traffic is the clearest possible sign that what you are watching is not reasoning about evidence. It is selection.

It may help to make this concrete. Suppose you encounter a claim that antiparasitic drugs shrink tumours, supported by a footnote to a real study. You open it. The study is in mice, using mebendazole, in a brain tumour model. Every word of it may be accurate.

Now list what it does not tell you. It does not tell you about ivermectin, which is a different chemical class. It does not tell you about fenbendazole, which is a related compound with entirely different absorption. It does not tell you about a person, because it was conducted in mice. It does not tell you about your cancer, unless your cancer is the one modelled. And it does not tell you what happened when mebendazole was subsequently tested in humans, which is in a different paper, and which was negative.

The footnote is real. The claim resting on it is several rungs and two compounds away from anything the paper established.

The transfer runs in a second direction too, and this one is more dangerous than the first.

People do not only borrow claims of benefit between these compounds. They borrow reassurance. Ivermectin has been given to hundreds of millions of people. Mebendazole has been approved for human use since the 1970s. Those facts are true, and they are frequently offered as grounds for confidence about all three, including the one with no human approval at all.

That inference has no basis. A safety record belongs to the compound that earned it. Fenbendazole's absorption, metabolism, and tolerability in people are not established, and the human reports that do exist describe liver injury. Nothing about ivermectin's public health record, and nothing about mebendazole's decades of approved use, says anything about what fenbendazole does in a human body.

Borrowing a claim of benefit costs you accuracy. Borrowing a claim of safety can cost you more than that.

WHEN THEY ARE TAKEN TOGETHER

Most people encountering these compounds are not considering one of them. Circulating protocols routinely combine two or three, often with supplements added.

This creates problems at every level.

Scientifically, a combination result describes the combination. The cohort study discussed above tested ivermectin and mebendazole together. Even if its data had been beyond question, it could not have told you what either compound contributed on its own, because no group received only one.

Practically, combinations multiply the interaction questions. Each additional compound is another thing for the liver to process. Each brings its own possible effects. Each is another candidate for an interaction with cancer treatment. Chapter 4 takes this up in detail, and it is the reason that chapter exists.

There is also a specific point about the liver worth flagging here, because it now appears in three separate places in this book. Published cases describe liver injury with fenbendazole. Trial data show liver enzyme elevations with mebendazole at oncology doses. The benzimidazole family more generally is associated with transient enzyme elevations during prolonged treatment. Now consider what a combination protocol does. It pairs two compounds from a family already associated with liver effects. It does so without monitoring. And it does so in a person whose liver may also be handling chemotherapy. That is not a neutral act. What that means for an individual is a question for a clinician, and Chapter 4 explains why it cannot be answered in a book.

Finally, combinations make personal accounts uninterpretable. When someone reports a good outcome on a three-compound protocol alongside conventional treatment, there are at least four candidate explanations and no way to separate them. The more elaborate the protocol, the less any individual outcome can tell you.

There is one more consequence of combining, and it runs against the intuition that drives it. The reasoning behind a multi-compound protocol is usually additive: if one might help, two might help more, and there is little to lose by including both. That reasoning treats potential benefits as stacking and potential harms as staying still.

Neither assumption is safe. Benefits do not automatically add; Chapter 2 described a study in which a compound combined with chemotherapy produced simply additive toxicity and no additional anticancer effect, which is a different and less appealing kind of addition. And harms genuinely can compound, particularly when two compounds are cleared through the same organ or produce the same side effect.

There is also a cost that is easy to overlook because it is not a side effect at all. A person taking four things cannot tell which one caused a problem. Neither can their oncologist. If something goes wrong, the safest response is usually to stop everything, including whatever might have been helping, and that includes the conventional treatment if the cause is unclear. Simplicity is not only easier. It preserves the ability to find out what is happening.

THREE VERDICTS, STATED SEPARATELY

The point of the last several thousand words is that these compounds require separate answers. Here they are.

Ivermectin. An approved human medicine with an excellent safety record at approved doses. Broad laboratory activity has been reported across many cancer types. Whether the concentrations at which that activity appears can be achieved in a person is genuinely disputed among researchers. It has entered human cancer trials. The first reported results come from a small dose-escalation study in which most evaluable patients progressed, and which was not designed to determine benefit. A larger randomised trial is planned. There is currently no evidence that it treats any cancer in humans, and the question is open in the specific sense that a study capable of answering it is now under way.

Mebendazole. An approved human medicine with decades of safety data at antiparasitic doses. It has the strongest and most reproduced preclinical case of the three, including evidence that it reaches brain tissue. It has been given to cancer patients in completed clinical trials. At oncology doses it caused significant liver enzyme elevations in some patients, reversible on stopping. In the one randomised trial published against a predefined benchmark, adding it to standard treatment for recurrent glioblastoma did not meet that benchmark. It is not approved for any cancer, and the strongest available human evidence is negative rather than absent.

Fenbendazole. Unchanged from the previous chapter. Veterinary only, no characterised human pharmacokinetics, no completed cancer trial, a retracted case series, and documented human cases of liver injury.

Notice that these three verdicts have different shapes. One is an open question with a trial running. One is a partly answered question where the answer was disappointing. One is a question nobody has yet asked properly. Anyone who tells you the same thing about all three has not read them.

Each verdict would also change under different conditions, and naming those conditions is what keeps this honest.

The ivermectin verdict would change if the planned randomised trial reported a benefit against a predefined endpoint, or if the concentration dispute were resolved in favour of achievability in patients. It would move the other way if that trial returned a negative result.

The mebendazole verdict would change if a randomised trial in a different cancer, or at an earlier stage, or in patients in better general condition, met a benchmark set in advance. The existing negative trial was in one difficult setting and does not close the whole question. It does mean that anyone claiming benefit now is claiming it against the best available evidence rather than in the absence of evidence.

The fenbendazole verdict would change if human pharmacokinetic data showed that meaningful concentrations are achievable, and if a trial followed. Neither exists.

Writing down what would change your mind is not a rhetorical flourish. It is the difference between a position and a commitment, and it is a reasonable thing to ask of anyone making claims in this area, including this book.

SIX QUESTIONS WORTH ASKING

These questions are about comparing evidence across compounds. They work on any claim in this area.

1. Which specific compound is this study about, and is it the one being recommended to me?

2. Was this study in cells, in animals, or in people? If in people, was there a comparison group?

3. If there was a benchmark set in advance, was it met?

4. Were participants taking anything else at the same time, and can the study separate the contributions?

5. Has this paper been corrected, questioned, or withdrawn since it was published?

6. If the strongest human evidence for one of these compounds is negative, what makes anyone confident about the others?

That last question is the one to carry with you. It is the question this chapter was built to make possible.

WHERE THIS LEADS

You now have the evidence, compound by compound.

What you do not yet have is the part that matters most for the person actually facing this decision. Every question in this chapter has been about whether these compounds work. None has been about what happens when a specific person takes one, in a body that is seventy-eight years old, on eight prescriptions, in the middle of chemotherapy, with a liver already doing more than usual.

That question has a different structure and it needs different tools.

It is also the question where the honest answer becomes least satisfying and most important. For most of what follows, the accurate response will be that nobody has studied it. That will be frustrating. It is also the single most useful thing a reader can know, because it tells you which questions to bring to a person who can look at your actual situation, rather than which article to read next.

Notice one more thing before moving on. Every safety observation in this chapter came from a setting where somebody was watching. The liver enzyme elevations in the mebendazole trial were found because investigators were testing for them. The side effects in the ivermectin study were recorded because recording them was the study's main purpose. That is what a trial is for, and it is the difference between a risk that gets caught and a risk that does not.

That difference is where the next chapter begins.

CHAPTER 4
SAFETY IS NOT A PROPERTY OF A COMPOUND

WHY "IS IT SAFE?" CANNOT BE ANSWERED

It is the most natural question in the world, and it is the wrong shape.

"Is fenbendazole safe?" sounds like it should have an answer, in the way that "is this water clean?" has an answer. But safety is not a property that a compound carries around with it. It is a relationship between a compound, an amount, a duration, a body, and everything else that body is doing at the time.

Change any one of those and the answer can change completely.

Consider a familiar example. Paracetamol, sold as Tylenol in the United States, is one of the safest medicines available. It is sold without a prescription and taken by millions of people every day. It is also a leading cause of acute liver failure. Both of those statements are true, and neither is surprising once you notice that they describe different amounts, different durations, and different livers.

So the question "is it safe?" has to be replaced. The useful version is longer and less satisfying: safe at what exposure, for how long, in whom, alongside what?

There is a term for the space between the amount that does something useful and the amount that causes harm. Pharmacologists call it the therapeutic window. Some drugs have a wide one, which is why they can be sold without a prescription. Others have a narrow one, which is why they are monitored carefully. Many cancer drugs fall into the second group.

For the compounds in this book, at oncology exposures, nobody knows where that window is. Not because it is narrow, and not because it is wide, but because establishing it requires the dose-finding studies described in Chapter 1, and those studies have not been done for fenbendazole and were only partly done for the other two.

This chapter is about that longer question. It will not tell you whether these compounds are safe for you, because that is not a question a book can answer. What it will do is show you the structure of the question, so that you know what has actually been studied, what has not, and which of the gaps matter for your situation.

Fair warning about what follows. For most of the specific questions in this chapter, the honest answer is that nobody has studied it. That is frustrating to read and it was frustrating to write. But there is a large practical difference between not knowing something and not knowing that you do not know it. The first is a position you can act from. The second is not.

WHAT THE PREVIOUS CHAPTERS ESTABLISHED, AND WHERE IT RUNS OUT

Chapter 3 ended on a principle: a safety record belongs to the compound and the exposure that earned it.

Everything in this chapter follows from taking that seriously.

Ivermectin's record comes from single doses or short courses, given to broadly healthy people, in public health programmes. Mebendazole's comes from short courses for intestinal worms. Fenbendazole has no human record at all, only published reports of harm.

Now look at what a cancer protocol asks of those records. It asks them to cover larger amounts, taken for months or years, by someone whose body is under strain, alongside treatments that place their own demands on the same organs. Not one of those extensions is supported by the data underneath the original record.

There is one place where the extension was actually tested, and it is instructive. When mebendazole was given at oncology exposures in a clinical trial, several patients developed significant liver enzyme elevations after about a month, and required dose reduction or discontinuation. Those patients were in a trial, being watched by investigators who were specifically looking for that. The signal appeared anyway [SRC-0033].

That is the single most useful data point in this chapter. It is not evidence that these compounds are dangerous. It is evidence that the approved-use safety record genuinely does not extend to oncology exposure, demonstrated in the one case where somebody checked.

AGE IS NOT THE VARIABLE THAT MATTERS

Before going further, something needs saying, because the rest of this chapter could easily be misread.

Nothing here is an argument that older adults should not ask these questions, or that they are too fragile to make their own decisions, or that their judgement needs supervision. Chronological age is not a diagnosis. Current professional guidance in cancer care says precisely this: the factors that matter, including physical function, other conditions, nutrition, cognition, and medication use, should be assessed in the individual rather than assumed from a date of birth [SRC-0006].

Two people of the same age can be entirely different patients. One runs, takes one prescription, and has excellent liver and kidney function. The other has three chronic conditions, takes ten medicines, and has kidneys working at half capacity. Age alone tells you almost nothing about which is which.

What age does reliably predict is not frailty. It is *variability*. Older populations are more spread out than younger ones on nearly every physiological measure. That is why individual assessment matters more with age, not less.

It is worth knowing what a proper assessment actually looks at, because it tells you what to ask for. The guidance describes several domains: how well someone moves and manages daily activities, what other medical conditions they have, how their thinking and memory are, their nutritional state, their mood, their social support, and their full medication list [SRC-0006]. Nothing in that list is age. Every item is something measurable about a particular person.

That distinction matters practically, and it cuts in the direction most readers will not expect. An assessment of this kind is not a mechanism for withholding treatment from older patients. It is frequently the opposite. It can identify a person who looks frail on paper but is in fact robust, and who can therefore be offered a treatment that a quick glance at their date of birth might have ruled out. It can also identify a specific fixable problem, such as poor nutrition or an unnecessary medication, that would otherwise have made treatment harder to tolerate.

So if you are an older adult reading this and wondering whether raising these questions will get you written off, the current professional guidance points the other way. Being assessed properly is how you avoid being assumed about.

There is also a documented reason why medication questions become more complicated over time. In a study of more than seven hundred adults aged seventy and over with advanced cancer starting a new treatment, sixty-one percent were taking five or more medicines and about fifteen percent were taking ten or more. Two-thirds were taking at least one medication considered potentially inappropriate for older adults. Non-prescription products, including vitamins and supplements, made up about a quarter of everything being taken, and accounted for a disproportionate share of the potentially inappropriate items. A quarter of patients had at least one potentially major drug interaction that did not even involve their cancer treatment. Each additional medication raised the odds of a major interaction by around forty percent [SRC-0007].

Read that last figure carefully, because it is the heart of this chapter. The risk does not come from any single item. It comes from the number of items and the connections between them. Adding one more thing to a list of ten is a different act from adding one more thing to a list of two.

Notice also that non-prescription products were doing more damage than their share of the list would suggest. The things people add themselves, without a prescription and often without mentioning them, were over-represented among the problems.

WHAT ACTUALLY CHANGES

The pharmacology here is not complicated, and knowing it changes how you read every claim about these compounds.

A drug's effect depends on how much of it is in the body and for how long. That depends on four things: how much gets absorbed, where it distributes, how it is broken down, and how it is removed. Ageing affects several of these, in ways that are well described.

Breakdown slows. Most drugs are processed by the liver, largely through a family of enzymes called cytochrome P450. Liver size and blood flow decline with age, and for drugs cleared this way, clearance typically falls by roughly a third [SRC-0039]. Slower clearance means a drug stays in the body longer. The same amount taken produces a higher accumulated exposure.

Removal slows. Kidney function declines steadily with age, even in people with no kidney disease. Drugs and their breakdown products that leave through the kidneys therefore leave more slowly [SRC-0039].

There is a detail here that surprises most people, including some clinicians. Kidney function is usually estimated from a blood test measuring creatinine, a waste product of muscle. Older adults typically have less muscle. Less muscle means less creatinine, which can make the estimate look better than the kidneys actually are [SRC-0039]. So a normal-looking result does not always mean normal function, and this is exactly the sort of thing a pharmacist or clinician can interpret and a website cannot.

Distribution changes. Body composition shifts with age: proportionally more fat, less water. Compounds that dissolve in fat spread into a larger reservoir and can linger. Compounds that dissolve in water are concentrated into a smaller one [SRC-0039]. This matters here, because these compounds are fat-soluble.

Protein binding changes. Many drugs travel through the blood attached to a protein called albumin, and only the unattached portion is active. Albumin levels tend to fall with age, and fall further with illness or poor nutrition. Less albumin can mean more unattached drug, which means more effect from the same amount [SRC-0039].

Absorption becomes less predictable. This one is less about age and more about the compounds themselves, but it compounds everything above. These are fat-soluble compounds, and how much of a fat-soluble compound gets absorbed depends considerably on what else is in the stomach at the time. Two people taking what they believe is an identical amount can end up with substantially different quantities in their bloodstream, simply because of when and with what they took it.

That is not a problem to be solved by adjusting anything. It is a reason the exposure is genuinely unknown. In a clinical trial this is handled by measuring blood levels, which is exactly what the mebendazole phase 1 study did, and it found levels varying considerably between patients even under controlled conditions [SRC-0033]. Outside a trial, nobody is measuring, and there is no way to know what a given person is actually receiving.

And kidneys matter more than people expect. The obvious point is that a compound and its breakdown products leave more slowly if the kidneys are working less well. The less obvious points are the ones that catch people out.

Kidney function is not fixed. It falls temporarily during illness, during dehydration, and after vomiting or diarrhoea, all of which are common during cancer treatment. A clearance that was adequate last month may not be adequate this week. This is why clinicians re-check rather than relying on an old result, and it is another reason a fixed protocol taken for months cannot account for what is happening in a particular body.

Several cancer treatments also place their own demands on the kidneys. Adding another substance to be cleared, in a person whose kidney function is already reduced by age and possibly further reduced by illness, is a question with no published answer for any of these compounds.

Now hold all four of those together and add one more fact from Chapter 2: the human pharmacokinetics of fenbendazole have never been characterised in anybody, at any age. The published work on how these compounds behave in an older body with cancer, over months, does not exist.

That is what the gap actually looks like. It is not that the answers are discouraging. It is that the questions have not been asked.

THE COMPLETE MEDICATION PICTURE

Almost every interaction question begins with an incomplete list, and incomplete lists are the norm rather than the exception.

The single most useful thing anyone can do here, before any decision is made, is assemble a genuinely complete picture of what is going into the body. Not a remembered list. A written one.

A complete medication picture includes:

- Every prescription medicine, with the name, the strength, and how often it is actually taken rather than how it was prescribed
- Every medicine bought without a prescription, including painkillers, antacids, sleep aids, and cold remedies
- Every vitamin, mineral, and supplement, including anything taken occasionally
- Every herbal or botanical product, including teas taken for a purpose
- Anything applied to the skin, inhaled, or used as drops
- Anything taken irregularly, such as a medicine used only when symptoms flare
- Anything recently stopped, and when
- Everything being taken from any protocol, named exactly
- Alcohol, and any recreational substance
- Any medicine prescribed by a different clinician who may not be in contact with the oncology team

That list is longer than most people expect, and it is meant to be. Two categories are missed almost every time. The first is anything the person does not think of as a medicine, which is where supplements, teas, and topical products disappear. The second is anything taken occasionally, because "I only take it sometimes" translates in memory to "I don't take it."

Assembling this is genuinely useful work. It is also work that does not require any medical knowledge, which makes it the single most valuable contribution a family member can make.

It is worth doing even if no decision about these compounds is pending. A complete, current list is useful at every appointment, in an emergency, and whenever a new prescription is added by anyone. Many people discover, on assembling it for the first time, that the list contains something they had forgotten about entirely, or two products containing the same active ingredient under different names.

One practical note. The most reliable way to build the list is not from memory. It is to physically gather every container in the house, including the ones in a bathroom cabinet, a bedside drawer, a handbag, and a kitchen shelf, and write down what is on each label.

It helps to know why each of the odder categories is on that list.

Occasional medicines matter because "occasional" is defined by the person, not by the body. A painkiller taken twice a week is a regular medicine. So is a sleep aid used on bad nights, and bad nights cluster during treatment.

Topical products matter because skin is not a barrier in the way people assume. Enough of some preparations is absorbed to have effects elsewhere.

Recently stopped medicines matter for the reason described above: the effect of a substance on a liver enzyme can persist for a week or two after the last dose.

Herbal teas matter when they are taken for a purpose rather than for pleasure. Something drunk daily for months to help with sleep or digestion is functioning as a medicine, whatever it is called.

And products from another prescriber matter because health systems are less joined-up than patients assume. A drug started by a cardiologist, a dermatologist, or a walk-in clinic may not appear on the oncology team's screen at all.

Write down the strength as well as the name. Two products with the same name can contain very different amounts, and the difference is exactly the sort of thing a pharmacist needs in order to be useful.

HOW INTERACTIONS ACTUALLY WORK

The phrase "drug interaction" covers two quite different things, and telling them apart is the most useful piece of pharmacology in this chapter.

The first kind changes how much of a drug is in the body. One substance interferes with how another is broken down or removed. The result is that the second drug's level goes up or down without anybody changing the amount taken.

The main site of this is that liver enzyme family, and particularly one member called CYP3A4, which is involved in processing roughly half of all medications [SRC-0040]. Substances that slow this enzyme cause other drugs to accumulate. Substances that speed it up cause them to be cleared faster. Grapefruit is a well-known example of the first, which is why it appears on so many medication warnings.

Now apply that to cancer treatment. Many oral cancer drugs are processed through exactly this pathway [SRC-0040]. That creates two distinct risks, and both matter.

If something slows the enzyme, a cancer drug can accumulate to levels that cause more side effects than intended. If something speeds it up, the cancer drug can be cleared too quickly, and the treatment may be less effective than the prescription implies.

Sit with that second possibility, because it is the one that almost never gets discussed. An interaction does not have to make you feel unwell to matter. It can quietly reduce the effectiveness of the treatment you are relying on, while producing no symptom at all. Nobody would notice until a scan.

The compounds in this book are relevant here. Fenbendazole is processed by liver enzymes including this one [SRC-0027]. Ivermectin is a substrate of the same enzyme, and known inhibitors of it can raise ivermectin levels. Mebendazole, at oncology exposures, produced liver enzyme elevations in trial patients [SRC-0033].

The second kind changes what the drugs do. Here the levels may be entirely normal. The problem is that two substances push in the same direction at once.

If two things each cause mild drowsiness, the combination may cause serious drowsiness. If two things each stress the liver a little, the combination may stress it a lot. No enzyme is involved and no level is abnormal. The effects simply add up.

This kind is easier to understand and easier to miss, because there is nothing to measure. It also does not require the two substances to be related in any way.

There is also a timing dimension that surprises people. Interactions do not always appear immediately and do not always disappear immediately. When a substance speeds up a liver enzyme, the body has to manufacture more of the enzyme, and the full effect typically takes ten days to two weeks to develop [SRC-0040]. The same applies in reverse when it is stopped.

The practical consequence is counterintuitive. Someone can start a compound, feel completely fine for a week, conclude that there is no interaction, and be wrong. And someone can stop a compound before an appointment, believing that this makes their disclosure unnecessary, while the effect on their treatment is still running.

That second scenario matters more than it sounds. "I stopped taking it" is not the same as "it is not affecting anything," and a clinician needs to know about a recent stop as much as a current use. This is why the medication picture below includes anything recently discontinued, with the date.

THE PUMP THAT PROTECTS YOUR BRAIN

There is one specific mechanism worth understanding in detail, because it illustrates the whole problem better than any general statement could.

Ivermectin is neurologically safe in humans for a specific reason. Your brain is protected by a barrier, and embedded in that barrier is a pump called P-glycoprotein. Its job is to catch certain substances that drift into the barrier cells and push them straight back out into the bloodstream. Ivermectin is one of the things it catches. Any that reaches the barrier gets ejected before it can enter the brain [SRC-0041].

That pump is the reason ivermectin can be given safely to hundreds of millions of people. It is not that ivermectin has no effect on nerve tissue. It is that it never gets there.

Now consider what could interfere with that arrangement. Researchers have identified several possibilities: unusually high exposures, genetic variations affecting the pump, disease that has damaged the barrier, and other drugs that compete for the same pump. Any of these could allow more ivermectin into the brain than normal [SRC-0041].

Look at that list again with a cancer patient in mind.

Cancer protocols involve exposures well above approved antiparasitic dosing. Cancer that has spread to the brain, or treatment directed at the brain, can compromise exactly the barrier in question. And a great many drugs, including several chemotherapy agents, interact with this same pump.

Now the irony, and it is a genuine one. One of the proposed anticancer mechanisms of ivermectin is that it interferes with a pump cancer cells use to expel drugs. That pump is P-glycoprotein. The very property being offered as a reason it might fight cancer is a property of the system that keeps it out of the brain.

Benzimidazoles interact with this transporter too, which means combination protocols involve more than one compound engaging the same system [SRC-0041].

It is worth noting who this does and does not apply to. For a healthy person taking an approved antiparasitic dose, the pump does its job and there is no issue; that is the basis of ivermectin's excellent public health record. The concern arises specifically where one or more of the listed conditions is present. A cancer patient on treatment, particularly one with disease affecting the brain, may have several of them at once.

That is a different situation from the one the safety record describes, which is the entire argument of this chapter arriving at a single concrete example.

Now here is the honest part. Nobody has studied whether this actually causes problems in cancer patients taking these compounds. There is no published series, no trial, no case-control study. What exists is a well-understood mechanism, a plausible route to harm, and a population in which several of the relevant conditions happen to be present at once.

That is not a warning that something bad will happen. It is a precise description of a question that has not been answered, and of why it cannot be answered by reading. Whether any of it applies to a particular person depends on that person's cancer, treatment, other medicines, and genetics. Those are things a clinician and a pharmacist can look at. They are not things a book can assess, and any source that tells you otherwise is selling something.

OVERLAPPING EFFECTS

Beyond formal interactions, there is a simpler problem: two things causing the same trouble.

Cancer treatment commonly causes fatigue, nausea, reduced appetite, and lowered blood counts. Liver enzyme changes are common during chemotherapy. Each of these is monitored, and each has an expected pattern that the oncology team knows how to interpret.

Now add a compound that can cause some of the same things. Benzimidazoles have been associated with liver enzyme elevations during prolonged treatment, and low blood counts were flagged as a concern in the mebendazole oncology trial [SRC-0033]. The published human reports for fenbendazole describe liver injury [SRC-0017].

Two consequences follow, and they are different.

The first is additive. If treatment stresses the liver a little and a compound stresses it a little, the total may exceed what either would produce alone.

The second is interpretive, and it is worse. When something goes wrong, nobody can tell where it came from.

Chapter 2 traced this sequence. An undisclosed compound causes liver injury. The injury is attributed to the chemotherapy or the immunotherapy, because that is the obvious suspect. The cancer treatment is paused, reduced, or abandoned. Sometimes immune-suppressing drugs are given for a problem that would have resolved on its own once the real cause was stopped.

The published case that required a formal structured causality assessment to untangle exists precisely because this is hard [SRC-0023]. Trained clinicians with the full picture found it difficult. Without the full picture, it is not difficult; it is impossible.

The cost of that misattribution is not the liver injury. It is the treatment that gets stopped.

There is a version of this problem that lands on the patient rather than the clinician, and it deserves its own attention because it is exhausting.

Suppose you are three months into treatment and taking a compound alongside it. You feel more tired than you did. Where did the tiredness come from? The cancer can cause it. The treatment causes it in most people. The compound might contribute. Poor sleep, worry, reduced appetite, and reduced activity all cause it too, and all of them are present.

You cannot answer that question by paying closer attention. Neither can anyone else, from the outside, with an incomplete list. And the natural response makes it worse: many people respond to a new symptom by adding something for it, which introduces another variable into a picture that already has too many.

This is the practical argument for keeping things simple that has nothing to do with whether any individual compound works. The fewer things you are doing at once, the more likely it is that anyone can tell what is happening to you. Interpretability is not a luxury during cancer treatment. It is how decisions get made about whether to continue, reduce, or change what you are receiving.

WHAT MONITORING CAN AND CANNOT DO

Protocol content often addresses safety concerns with a reassuring phrase: just get your liver checked.

It is worth understanding precisely what that does and does not accomplish.

Blood tests can detect certain kinds of damage after they have begun. Liver enzyme elevations show that liver cells have been injured. Blood counts show that the marrow is under strain. These are genuinely useful, which is why they are used in trials and in ordinary care.

Here is what they cannot do.

They cannot tell you *what* caused the change. A raised liver enzyme is a signal, not an explanation. Distinguishing a compound from chemotherapy from the cancer itself requires clinical judgement, timing information, and often a formal assessment.

They cannot detect problems in tissues they do not measure. A liver panel says nothing about the nervous system, the heart, or the kidneys.

They cannot detect an interaction that is reducing the effectiveness of your cancer treatment. There is no blood test for "your chemotherapy is being cleared faster than intended." That would show up months later, on a scan, as a treatment that did not work as well as expected.

And most importantly, they cannot prevent anything. Monitoring detects harm that has already started. Whether that is early enough depends entirely on how fast the harm develops and on how the results are interpreted, which is a clinical matter.

Notice what all of this implies. Every genuine protection here depends on somebody who knows the full situation looking at the results. Testing without that is not a safety measure. It is data collection.

It is worth being precise about what a clinical trial provides that testing on your own does not, because the difference is not the blood test. It is everything around it.

A trial has stopping rules written down before anyone enrols: what result triggers a dose reduction, what result triggers stopping altogether, and who decides. It has somebody whose job is to look at each result promptly rather than when they next have time. It has a defined schedule tied to what is known about how the compound behaves. And it has a mechanism for recording what happened, so that the next patient benefits from it.

The mebendazole trial in Chapter 3 illustrates all of this. Four patients developed significant liver enzyme elevations. Those were detected, acted upon, reversed, and published. That sequence is what a trial is. Remove the investigators, the pre-written rules, and the reporting, and you are left with a blood test and a person hoping they will know what to do with the number.

This is also why this book does not tell you what to monitor or how often. Not out of caution, but because a monitoring plan is a clinical decision that depends on the person, the treatment, the compound, and the exposure. Any schedule offered by a website is being made up, and a plan made up is not a safeguard. It is the appearance of one.

WHAT "UNSTUDIED" ACTUALLY MEANS

This chapter has used the word *unstudied* many times, and it is worth separating what it means from what it is often taken to mean.

There are three quite different situations that people collapse into one.

Somebody looked and found nothing. A study was designed to detect an interaction, it was adequately sized, and it found none. This is genuine reassurance, bounded by the study's design and population.

Somebody looked and found something. An interaction is documented and appears in prescribing information, where clinicians and pharmacists can check it.

Nobody looked. No study exists. Nothing is known in either direction.

The phrase "no known interaction" is used for all three, and this is the most consequential ambiguity in the whole subject. For fenbendazole with any cancer treatment, the accurate statement is the third. It is not that studies have looked and found the combination safe. It is that the question has not been asked.

Chapter 1 insisted on this distinction and it applies with full force here. Absence of evidence about an interaction is not evidence that there is no interaction. It is also not evidence that there is one. It is a blank space, and it should be described as a blank space rather than filled in by whichever assumption the reader prefers.

This has a direct practical implication, and it is the reason a pharmacist is worth more than a search engine here. Interaction-checking tools work by looking up documented pairs in a database. If you enter a compound that has never been formally studied, the tool will return nothing, and nothing looks exactly like reassurance. It is not. It is the tool reporting that it has no entry.

A pharmacist reading the same blank space sees something different. They can reason from what the compound is chemically, which enzymes and transporters it is likely to engage, and what else the person is taking. That reasoning does not produce certainty. It produces something considerably more useful than a database returning no results.

WHY "NATURAL" AND "WELL TOLERATED" MISLEAD HERE

Two reassuring words do a great deal of work in this area, and neither means what it appears to.

Natural is not a claim about safety. It is a claim about origin, and origin does not predict effect. A great many potent toxins are entirely natural, and several important chemotherapy drugs were originally derived from plants. In any case, the compounds in this book are not natural in any ordinary sense. They are manufactured pharmaceuticals, synthesised in factories, and the fact that one of them is sold for animals does not make it closer to nature.

Well tolerated is a real term with a specific meaning, and the meaning is bounded. It means that in the studied population, at the studied exposure, for the studied duration, most people did not experience unacceptable side effects. Strip away those three qualifiers and the phrase becomes meaningless.

Chapter 2 examined what one such record consists of: twenty-eight healthy cats, nine days. That study was well conducted and it is genuinely reassuring about the thing it examined. It says nothing about a person taking the same compound for a year during chemotherapy.

There is a third reassurance worth naming, because it is subtler. People often reason that if a compound has been used for decades without problems being reported, problems must be rare.

That inference requires somebody to be counting. For approved medicines used as approved, somebody is: adverse events are recorded and there are reporting systems. For a compound taken privately, outside medical care, and frequently not mentioned to anyone, nobody is counting. Harm surfaces only when a person becomes unwell enough to reach a hospital and a clinician thinks to ask the right question. The published cases in this book are, by definition, the ones that got that far.

That does not mean harm is common. It means the absence of reports is not a measurement, and it should not be read as one.

Where a Family Member Can Actually Help

This is a chapter about complexity, and complexity is where an extra person is most useful. But the useful role is narrower and more concrete than most families assume.

Here is what genuinely helps.

Assembling the complete medication picture. Gathering every container in the house and writing down what is on each label. This requires no medical knowledge and it is the foundation for every other question in this chapter.

Keeping a timeline. When something started, when a dose changed, when a symptom appeared. Timing is central to working out whether a compound caused a problem, and it is precisely the information that is hardest to reconstruct afterwards.

Holding the sources. The link, the date, the name of the study, whatever was actually claimed.

Being at the appointment. Two people hear more than one, especially when one of them has just received difficult news.

Writing down what was said. Not what it felt like. What was said.

Now the harder part.

None of this includes deciding. The person whose body it is holds that decision, even when a family member is better informed, even when the family member disagrees, and even when the decision looks like a mistake. A caregiver who takes over the decision has not protected anyone. They have removed the only person with standing to make it.

There is a specific version of this worth naming, because it happens often. A family member finds this material, becomes convinced, and starts pressing. The pressure is loving and it is exhausting to receive. Someone with cancer already has a great deal to manage, and defending a decision at the kitchen table is a cost they should not have to bear on top of everything else.

The useful question is not "have you considered this?" repeated in different forms. It is "how much do you want to know, and how involved do you want me to be?" Then acting on the answer, including when the answer is *less*.

There is a harder version of this, and pretending otherwise would be dishonest. Sometimes a family member is convinced that a compound will help and the patient is not interested. Sometimes it runs the other way: the patient wants to try something and the family is frightened by it.

Neither situation is resolved by winning the argument, and both are made worse by conducting it repeatedly.

What can help is separating the two things that get tangled together. One is the evidence, which is a factual matter and which this book has tried to set out. The other is the decision, which is not purely factual and which belongs to one person. Two people can agree completely about what the evidence shows and still disagree about what to do, because they weigh uncertainty differently, and that difference is legitimate.

If you are the family member, the most useful sentence you have is often not an argument at all. It is an offer: to write down the questions, to come to the appointment, to keep the list. That contribution is real, it is needed, and it does not require anyone to change their mind.

One more practical point. If you are attending an appointment on someone's behalf or alongside them, ask beforehand what they want raised and what they do not. Arriving with a list of concerns the patient did not agree to is a common way for a well-intentioned family member to make an appointment worse.

Living With an Honest Answer

Most of this chapter has consisted of saying that something has not been studied. It would be reasonable to reach this point feeling that you have learned nothing useful.

You have, and it is worth naming what.

You now know which questions have answers and which do not. You know that the safety record does not extend to oncology exposure, and that this was demonstrated the one time it was checked. You know that interactions come in two kinds, and that one of them can quietly weaken your treatment without producing a symptom. You know that a specific mechanism exists by which one of these compounds could reach the brain in circumstances a cancer patient might plausibly be in, and that nobody has studied whether it does. You know what monitoring can and cannot detect, and why a schedule from a website is not a safeguard.

That is not nothing. It is the difference between a vague sense that something might be risky and a specific list of things to ask about.

There is one more thing worth saying about deciding under this kind of uncertainty, and it is not a recommendation in either direction.

Decisions differ in how easily they can be undone. Some choices can be reversed if they turn out badly; others cannot. That distinction is often more useful than trying to settle an unanswerable question about whether something works. It also suggests an obvious sequence: the questions that could change your decision are worth asking before you act, not afterwards, because information arriving afterwards has fewer options left to work with.

It is also worth noticing that the choice is rarely as binary as it feels at three in the morning. Between doing nothing and starting something privately there are several other options, including asking whether a trial exists that you would be eligible for, asking a pharmacist to look at your specific list before anything changes, and asking your oncologist directly what they would want to know if you did go ahead. None of those forecloses anything.

What this book cannot do is tell you what to weigh more heavily. People facing the same evidence reasonably reach different conclusions, depending on what they are willing to risk and what they are hoping for. That is not a failure of reasoning. It is what deciding under uncertainty is.

Here is the table that summarises it.

Factor	Why it matters	What is known	Who can answer it
Exposure and duration	Safety records cover short courses; protocols run for months	Approved-use data do not extend; the one oncology trial found liver enzyme elevations	Oncology team, pharmacist
Liver function	Most breakdown happens here; cancer treatment loads the same organ	Human liver injury reported with fenbendazole; enzyme elevations with mebendazole at oncology doses	Oncology team, pharmacist
Kidney function	Governs removal; declines with age and can be overestimated by routine tests	Not studied for these compounds in this population	Clinician, pharmacist
Metabolic interactions	Can raise or lower the level of your cancer treatment	Shared enzyme pathways involved; specific effects unstudied	Pharmacist, oncology team
Transporter interactions	Governs what reaches the brain and what tumours expel	Mechanism well described; consequences in cancer patients unstudied	Oncology team
Overlapping side effects	Two causes of the same problem become impossible to separate	Documented for liver effects and blood counts	Oncology team
Other medicines	Each addition raises interaction odds substantially	Well established in older adults with cancer	Pharmacist
Your specific situation	Everything above depends on it	Nothing in any book	Only your clinicians

Look down the third column. Most of it says unstudied. Now look down the fourth. Every row has somebody in it.

That is the actual finding of this chapter. The uncertainty is real and it is not going to be resolved by more reading. But every unanswered question has a person attached to it who can at least look at your version of it.

EIGHT QUESTIONS WORTH ASKING

These are for the oncology team, and several are specifically for a pharmacist, who is often the most accessible and most underused person in the whole system.

1. Here is my complete list, including supplements and anything I take occasionally. Is there anything on it that concerns you?
2. Is my cancer treatment processed by the liver in a way that something else could speed up or slow down?
3. If something interfered with my treatment's effectiveness rather than causing side effects, how would we find out, and when?
4. Given my liver and kidney function specifically, is there anything about how I clear medicines that I should understand?
5. If I developed a problem, how would you work out whether it came from my treatment or from something else I was taking?
6. Are there side effects my treatment causes that something else might add to?
7. Is there anything about my cancer or my treatment that affects the barrier protecting my brain?
8. If I decide to take something you would not recommend, what would you want to know, and how would you want me to tell you?

That last question is the important one, and it is worth saying why once more. Chapter 2 described what happens when a compound is taken without disclosure: harm gets attributed to the cancer treatment, and the treatment is stopped.

The evidence says this is the normal case, not the exception. Reviews of studies covering cancer patients found that between a fifth and three-quarters of those using complementary approaches did not tell their doctors [SRC-0042]. The reasons are consistent and worth reading, because they are probably yours. The doctor never asked. The patient expected disapproval, or disinterest, or that the doctor would not be able to help. Or the patient assumed it was simply not relevant to their conventional care [SRC-0042].

Every one of those is understandable. The last one is the most consequential, because this chapter has been an extended demonstration that it is not true.

You are allowed to disagree with your oncologist. You are allowed to make a decision they would not make. What you cannot do, without cost, is leave them working from an incomplete picture, because the picture is the only tool they have for telling one problem from another.

IF YOU ARE ALREADY TAKING SOMETHING

A good number of people reading this chapter will not be deciding whether to start. They will already have started, possibly months ago, and possibly without telling anyone.

If that is you, the questions in this chapter still apply, but their shape changes.

The first thing worth saying is that nothing here is an argument for panic. Most of the reported human harms in this book developed over weeks to months and resolved once the compound was stopped. That is a description of what has been published, not a prediction about you, and it is not a reason to relax either. It is a reason to act deliberately rather than urgently.

The second is that the disclosure conversation is different, and in one respect easier. You are not asking permission for something. You are providing information about something that is already happening, which is a considerably simpler thing to say. Clinicians hear this more often than most patients imagine, and the evidence in this chapter suggests they suspect it more often than they say.

Three things are worth bringing to that conversation. What you have been taking, named exactly, including anything alongside it. When you started, and whether the amount has changed at any point. And whether anything has felt different since, even if it seemed unrelated at the time.

That third item is where people leave out the most. A change in energy, appetite, sleep, or digestion feels like part of having cancer, and it usually is. But it is not your job to work out which changes are relevant. Reporting them is what makes it possible for someone else to do that.

One more thing worth knowing. If you decide to stop something, that is worth mentioning too, and worth dating. As this chapter explained, effects on liver enzymes can persist for a week or two after the last dose, so a recent stop is still clinically relevant. "I was taking it until three weeks ago" is useful information. Saying nothing because you have stopped is not the same as the question having gone away.

WHERE THIS LEADS

Every question in this chapter routes to the same place: a conversation with someone who can see your actual situation.

That conversation is not always easy to have. There is limited time. There is a real fear of being judged, or dismissed, or of damaging a relationship you depend on. There may have been a previous attempt that did not go well.

So the remaining question is a practical one. How do you turn everything you have worked out into a conversation that produces answers, in fifteen minutes, with someone you may be nervous about disappointing?

There is one thing to carry into it. Everything in this chapter has been about a question that only exists in the plural. Not "is this safe" but "is this safe for me, at this exposure, for this long, alongside these eight other things."

No article answers that question. No forum answers it. This book does not answer it. Only somebody looking at your actual situation can, and that is not a limitation of the material. It is the finding.

That is where the next chapter begins.

CHAPTER 5
TURNING WHAT YOU KNOW INTO A CONVERSATION

THE ONLY PLACE THIS CAN BE SETTLED

Everything in this book has been building toward a room with two people in it and not much time.

That is not a disappointing ending. It is the honest one. Chapter 4 showed that every question worth asking about these compounds depends on facts about a particular person: their cancer, their treatment, their liver, their kidneys, their other medicines. Those facts are not in any article, and no amount of further reading will produce them.

So the remaining work is practical. How do you take what you have worked out and turn it into fifteen minutes that actually produces answers?

The obstacles are real and worth naming. Appointments are short. You may be tired, or frightened, or still absorbing something you were told at the start of the visit. You may worry about being judged, or about damaging a relationship you depend on. You may have tried before and had it go badly.

None of that is solved by being told to communicate better. What helps is preparation, and preparation is something you can do in advance, on a good day, at your kitchen table.

This chapter is about that preparation. It is not about persuasion. Nothing here is designed to talk a clinician into anything, and a chapter that did that would be doing you a disservice. The goal is a conversation where you learn something you did not know, which is a different and more achievable target.

It also helps to be realistic about what is on the other side of the desk.

Your oncologist knows things you cannot look up. They know your disease and its behaviour, your scans, your pathology, how you have responded so far, and what the plan depends on. That knowledge is the reason this conversation is worth having.

They may also not know much about the specific compound you want to ask about. That is not a failure. Nobody can be current on every substance circulating online, and as Chapters 2 and 3 showed, the published evidence for these compounds is thin, scattered, and in two cases carries integrity notices. A clinician who says they are not familiar with the details is being accurate.

What they can do, reliably, is the thing that actually matters: look at your treatment, your organ function, and your medication list, and tell you what they can see from there. If you arrive expecting a verdict on the compound, you may be disappointed. If you arrive with a question about your situation, you will get something useful.

There is also the matter of time. A typical appointment is short and much of it is already spoken for. This is not indifference; it is how the system is built. Preparation is how you get your question into the part of the visit that remains.

FREEZING THE CLAIM

The first step happens long before the appointment, and it takes about a minute.

When you encounter a claim you want to ask about, save it immediately. The link, the date you found it, and a screenshot if it is a post that might disappear. If it is a video, note the title, the channel, and roughly where in it the claim appears.

This sounds fussy. It is the difference between a conversation that goes somewhere and one that does not.

Claims degrade as they travel. The version you read may have already lost the qualifications the original author included. By the time you are sitting in front of your oncologist, trying to reconstruct it from memory, it will have degraded again. "I read something about a dewormer that cures cancer" is not a question anybody can answer. It invites a general response, which is what it deserves, and then everyone moves on.

There is a second reason, which Chapters 2 and 3 demonstrated. A source's status can change after you read it. One prominent case series was retracted. One widely cited cohort study now carries an Expression of Concern. If you saved the citation, you can check. If you remembered the gist, you cannot.

If somebody else sent you the claim, ask them for the original source rather than their summary of it. If they cannot produce one, that is already useful information.

THE CLAIM BRIEF

Once you have the source, condense it onto one page. This is the single most useful document you can bring, and it takes fifteen minutes to make.

A claim brief has seven parts.

The claim, in one sentence. Written as an assertion, with the story stripped out. Not "there's a lot of talk about fenbendazole." Rather: "This compound produced tumour shrinkage in patients with this cancer."

The compound, named exactly. Which one. Human medicine or veterinary product. If a specific preparation is involved, say so.

Where you found it. The source, with the date you found it.

What the underlying evidence is, if you could find it. Cells, animals, one person, a group of people, or a trial. If the claim cited a study, name it. If it cited nothing, write that down, because it is the most important thing on the page.

What you already checked. Whether the paper has a notice attached. Whether the study was in the same compound the claim is about. This shows you have done work, which changes how the conversation goes.

Your specific question. Not "what do you think?" Something answerable.

What you are actually considering. Whether you are asking out of curiosity, or seriously thinking about taking it, or already taking it. This matters more than anything else on the page, and it is the part people most often leave out.

That last item deserves emphasis. A clinician answers a curiosity question differently from a decision question, and they should. If you are already taking something, say so at the start rather than working up to it. Chapter 4 explained why: the information changes what they are able to do for you.

Keep the brief to one page. If it runs longer, you are including the story rather than the claim.

Here is what a completed brief looks like. The details are invented; the shape is the point.

Claim: Taking this compound alongside chemotherapy shrinks tumours in people with my cancer type.

>

Compound: Fenbendazole. Veterinary product, no human formulation.

>

Source: Video, found 14 March. Channel and link saved on my phone.

>

Evidence cited: One study, in mice, from 2018. The video did not mention any human trial.

>

What I checked: The 2018 study is real and is in mice. I could not find a completed human trial. One case series on this compound was retracted in January 2026.

>

My question: I am on treatment that I think is processed by the liver. If I took something else processed the same way, could that change how well my treatment works?

>

Where I stand: Seriously considering it. Not taking it yet.

Notice what that page does. It takes under a minute to read. It shows that you have already separated the claim from the story and located the evidence. It asks something answerable. And it tells the clinician exactly what is at stake, which determines how much of the remaining time they should spend on it.

Notice also what it does not do. It does not argue. It does not ask anyone to agree. It contains no persuasion at all, and it is more likely to produce a real answer because of that.

WHAT ELSE TO BRING

Chapter 4 described the complete medication picture. Bring it, written down, on paper.

Two practical notes. Bring a copy you can leave behind, because a list that goes home in your bag is a list nobody can check later. And write the date on it, because it will be out of date within months and a stale list read as current is worse than none.

Bring one other thing: a short written list of your questions, in priority order. Appointments get derailed. Scan results arrive. Something unexpected comes up. If your questions exist only in your head, the ones at the bottom will not survive the visit. If they are on paper, you can hand the paper over.

QUESTIONS THAT PRODUCE ANSWERS

There is a pattern to questions that work and questions that do not, and it is easy to learn.

Questions that invite a general answer get one. "What do you think about fenbendazole?" is a request for an opinion, and a busy clinician will give you a short one. It will probably be accurate and it will probably not tell you anything you did not already know.

Questions anchored to something specific produce specific answers. The anchor can be a study, a compound, your treatment, or your own body. Here is the difference in practice.

Instead of asking	Ask
What do you think about these antiparasitic drugs?	Is there anything in my current treatment that could interact with a compound processed by liver enzymes?
Is fenbendazole safe?	If I took something and my liver tests changed, how would you work out what caused it?
Have you seen the studies on this?	This study was in mice, with a different compound. Is there anything in it that would apply to my situation?
Does it work?	Is there a trial of any of these compounds I would be eligible for?

Instead of asking	Ask
Are you against alternative treatments?	If I decided to take something you would not recommend, what would you want to know, and how would you want me to tell you?
Why isn't anyone researching cheap drugs?	Who would I talk to about whether a compound like this is worth studying in my cancer?

Look at the right-hand column. Every question has an anchor and none is a challenge. That is not about being polite. A question phrased as a challenge produces a defensive answer, and a defensive answer contains less information. You are not trying to win. You are trying to find something out.

Write the answers down during the appointment, or have someone with you who can. This is not about mistrust. People retain remarkably little from a medical conversation, and that is true of everyone, particularly when the visit began with news. An answer you half-remember is an answer you will end up re-litigating on the internet at midnight.

If you can, bring someone. Two people hear more than one, and the second person can write while the first listens. Agree beforehand on what will be raised, so that nobody is surprised.

Some clinics allow you to record the conversation. Ask first; policies vary and asking is the whole of the etiquette.

One more thing worth doing. When you get an answer, repeat it back in your own words and ask whether you have understood. This is not a courtesy. It is the fastest way to catch the misunderstanding that would otherwise send you home with a wrong idea, and clinicians generally welcome it because it is how they find out what actually landed.

WHEN THE ANSWER IS "I DON'T KNOW"

For many questions in this book, that is the correct answer, and you should expect to hear it.

It is worth recognising it as a good sign rather than a failure. A clinician who says they do not know whether a compound with no published human pharmacokinetics will interact with your treatment is telling you the truth. Someone who answers that question confidently, in either direction, is telling you something they cannot know.

But "I don't know" is a starting point, not an ending, and there are three useful follow-ups.

"Is that unknown for everyone, or unknown for my situation specifically?" This separates a gap in the science from a gap in what can be determined about you. They are different problems with different next steps.

"Is there someone who would know more?" Usually a pharmacist. Sometimes a specialist service. Asking this converts a dead end into a referral.

"What would you want to happen if I went ahead anyway?" This is the question that keeps the door open. It produces practical information regardless of what anyone thinks of the underlying idea, and it makes clear that you are not asking for endorsement.

Chapter 4 explained why an unstudied question is not the same as a settled one. This is where that distinction becomes useful rather than merely accurate.

WHEN IT GOES BADLY

Sometimes it does, and pretending otherwise would be useless.

You may be dismissed. You may get a one-line answer that closes the subject. You may be told not to believe things you read online, in a tone that suggests the conversation is over. You may sense disapproval and decide not to mention the rest.

First, what this usually is. Clinicians in this field encounter these questions constantly, often from people who have already decided, and often in a form that is hostile. Some have watched patients delay effective treatment. That history shapes how they hear the topic before you have finished your sentence. It is not usually about you.

That explanation is not a justification, and being dismissed is a poor outcome regardless of its cause. But knowing what you are dealing with makes the next step easier to choose.

Several things can help.

Lead with the medication picture rather than the claim. "Here is everything I am taking, including things I have added myself. Is there anything here that concerns you?" is a different conversation from "what do you think about this drug I read about." It is also more useful, because it is the question with the more important answer.

Name what you are asking for. "I am not asking you to prescribe anything. I want to understand whether this could interfere with my treatment." That single sentence removes the fear that is usually driving the defensiveness.

Ask the narrow question. A broad question invites a broad dismissal. A narrow one is harder to wave away and easier to answer.

Try a different member of the team. A pharmacist, an oncology nurse, or a nurse navigator may have more time and a different relationship to the question. This is not going behind anyone's back. It is using the team.

Ask for it to be written in your notes. "Could you note that I raised this?" is a reasonable request. It creates a record, and records are useful later.

Now the thing this chapter will not do.

If a clinician tells you they would not recommend something, that is an answer, and it is not an invitation to keep asking until somebody says yes. There is a genuine difference between seeking a second opinion, which is legitimate and covered below, and continuing until you find a prescriber who agrees. The first is about information. The second is about obtaining a result, and it is how people end up in the hands of the operators described at the end of this chapter.

If the relationship has broken down beyond repair, that is a different problem with a legitimate solution, which is changing clinicians through the ordinary route. It is not solved by concealment.

There is a harder version of this situation, and it is common enough to address directly.

Suppose you are already taking something and have not said so, and now you are afraid to. The longer it goes on, the harder it gets, and the fear compounds: not just of disapproval, but of having to explain why you did not mention it sooner.

Two things are worth knowing.

The first is that this is the normal case, not an unusual lapse. The evidence in Chapter 4 found that a substantial proportion of cancer patients using complementary approaches do not tell their doctors, and that one of the commonest reasons is simply that nobody asked [SRC-0042]. You are not confessing to something rare.

The second is that the conversation does not require an explanation. "There is something I have been taking that I have not mentioned" is a complete opening. You do not owe anyone an account of your reasoning, and most clinicians will move straight to the practical question, because that is the part they can act on.

If saying it aloud feels impossible, write it on the medication list and hand the list over. It is on the record, which is what matters.

WHO CAN HELP WITH WHAT

Most people bring every question to their oncologist, who has the least time of anyone involved. The team is larger than that, and different members can answer different things.

Who	Best for	Not the right person for
Medical oncologist	Your treatment plan, prognosis, whether something could interfere, trial eligibility	Detailed interaction checking; long conversations about a specific paper
Oncology pharmacist	Interactions, your full medication list, how compounds are processed, what a database can and cannot tell you	Decisions about your cancer treatment
Oncology nurse or nurse navigator	What to expect, what to report and when, how to get questions answered between visits, navigating the system	Prescribing or changing treatment
General practitioner	Your other conditions and medicines, coordination, the whole picture over time	Specialist decisions about your cancer
Palliative care team	Symptoms, side effects, quality of life, complex decisions, support for the family	Nothing you should hesitate to raise with them
Clinical trial team	What a specific trial involves, eligibility, what participation would mean	Advice about anything outside the trial

Two entries deserve expanding.

The pharmacist is the most underused person in this list. Interaction questions are their core expertise, they usually have more time than the oncologist, and Chapter 4 explained why they can do something an interaction-checking website cannot. A database returns nothing for a compound that has never been studied, and nothing looks like reassurance. A pharmacist reading the same blank space can reason from what the compound is chemically, which systems it is likely to engage, and what else you are taking. Many cancer centres have a pharmacist available, and in most systems you can simply ask to speak to one.

Palliative care is not what most people think it is. It is routinely confused with end-of-life care, and that confusion costs people a great deal. Palliative care is specialised support focused on symptoms, side effects, and quality of life, provided alongside active treatment rather than instead of it.

The evidence on this is unusually strong. A randomised trial in patients with metastatic lung cancer found that introducing palliative care early, alongside standard treatment, improved quality of life and mood [SRC-0047]. Current professional guidance recommends that people with advanced cancer receive it early in the course of illness, concurrently with active treatment, rather than in the final weeks [SRC-0046].

If you are struggling with side effects, or with the sheer weight of managing all this, a palliative care referral is one of the most evidence-based things available, and asking for one is not giving up on anything.

There is a specific reason it belongs in this chapter. Palliative care teams tend to have longer appointments than oncology clinics, and their remit explicitly includes complex decisions and the family's questions as well as the patient's. If the conversation this chapter describes keeps failing to fit into a fifteen-minute slot, that is often where it fits.

A note on the caregiver's role in the room. Chapter 4 described the organisational work. In the appointment itself, the useful role is narrower still: take notes, keep the question list visible, and prompt if something on it has been missed.

What does not help is answering on the patient's behalf, or raising items they did not agree to. Both are common and both shift the conversation away from the person it is about. Agree beforehand what you will raise and what you will leave alone, and stick to it even if you disagree.

SECOND OPINIONS

A second opinion is a normal part of cancer care. Clinicians expect them, most are not offended, and in many systems they are straightforward to arrange.

What a second opinion is for: confirming a diagnosis, reviewing whether the treatment plan is the one another specialist would choose, identifying options or trials available elsewhere, and getting a fresh explanation when the first one did not land.

What it is not for: finding someone who will say yes to something the first clinician declined.

The distinction matters more than it might seem. A genuine second opinion involves a qualified specialist reviewing your actual records, imaging, and pathology, and reaching their own conclusion. That is valuable even when it confirms what you were already told, because confirmation from an independent source is information.

Practical points. Ask your team to send your records rather than carrying an incomplete set yourself; a specialist reviewing partial information is not giving you a second opinion, they are guessing. Large cancer centres often have formal second-opinion services, sometimes remotely. And a second opinion is most useful at a decision point, before a course of treatment begins, rather than partway through.

Telling your current team is the norm, not a betrayal. Most will help arrange it.

If a second opinion is difficult to arrange where you are, a few things still help. Some large centres offer remote record reviews. Some cancers have specialist centres that will comment on a case without you travelling. And in some systems a general practitioner can request a specialist review on your behalf when a direct request has stalled.

If none of that is available, the fallback is narrower but still worth having: ask your own team to explain the reasoning behind the plan, including what the alternatives were and why they were not chosen. That is not a second opinion. It is often most of what people were hoping a second opinion would give them.

BETWEEN APPOINTMENTS

Most of this chapter concerns a single conversation. Most of what happens, happens in the weeks between them.

It is worth establishing, in advance, how to reach your team and what they want to hear about. Not what you should watch for; that is a clinical judgement and it belongs to them. What you want is the channel and the threshold, in their words.

Useful questions to settle early: Who do I contact between visits, and how? Is there a nurse line, and what are its hours? What would you want to hear about promptly rather than at my next appointment? And where do I go outside those hours?

Write the answers somewhere findable, and make sure whoever is helping you knows where that is. The moment you need this information is exactly the moment nobody can think clearly enough to look for it.

Two things are worth reporting even when they feel unrelated. Anything you started or stopped taking, including things you added yourself. And any change you noticed that you cannot explain, even if you suspect it is nothing. Chapter 4 explained why: you are not expected to work out what is relevant. Reporting it is what allows someone else to.

Keep a simple running note of dates. When something started, when it changed, when a symptom appeared. It takes seconds at the time and is impossible to reconstruct months later, and timing is central to working out what caused what.

CLINICAL TRIALS

Chapter 3 mentioned a planned randomised trial of one of these compounds. Trials in general are worth understanding, because they are the legitimate route to an investigational treatment and most people never look.

The main public listing in the United States is maintained by the National Cancer Institute and covers cancer trials specifically, with a search designed for patients rather than researchers [SRC-0045]. The broader government registry described in Chapter 1 lists trials across all conditions.

A few things to understand before you look.

A listing is not a recommendation. Chapter 1 made this point and it bears repeating. Registration is a legal requirement triggered by a study starting. It says a question is being asked, not that anyone expects a particular answer.

Eligibility criteria are strict and they are not personal. Trials specify cancer type, stage, previous treatments, organ function, and other requirements. These exist so that the results mean something. Being ineligible is common and is not a judgement about you.

Phase tells you what the trial is for. An early-phase trial is primarily establishing safety and dosing. A later-phase trial is testing whether something works better than the alternative. Both are legitimate; they answer different questions, and you should know which one you would be joining.

Ask what participation actually involves. How often you would attend, what extra tests are required, how far you would travel, what happens if you want to stop, and what happens to your care afterwards.

Ask what you would receive. In a randomised trial you may receive the comparison treatment rather than the new one, and the comparison is usually the current standard rather than nothing.

Your oncologist is the right person to start with, because they know your situation and can often identify trials you would not find. A search is a good preparation for that conversation rather than a substitute for it.

Ask what informed consent involves. You will be given a document describing the trial, its risks, what is known and unknown, and your right to withdraw at any time without affecting your other care. Take it home. Read it somewhere quiet. Bring questions back. Nobody should be asking you to sign it in the room, and a well-run trial will expect you to take your time.

There is also a legitimate pathway outside trials that most people have never heard of. Regulators operate a mechanism sometimes called expanded access, through which a patient may in defined circumstances receive an investigational drug outside a study, when no comparable option exists and they cannot enrol in a trial. It is not available for every compound, it requires a physician to initiate it, and it is subject to regulatory and ethical approval [SRC-0011].

The reason to mention it is not that it applies to the compounds in this book. It is that a route exists, it is regulated, it involves your own doctor, and knowing it exists makes it easier to recognise what is not it.

One caution follows directly. Some organisations describe themselves as offering access to investigational treatments outside a formal trial, sometimes for a fee. A genuine clinical trial does not charge you for the investigational treatment, and a legitimate expanded-access request goes through your physician and a regulator, not through a payment page. That is one of the clearest lines available, and it leads directly to the last section.

WARNING SIGNS

A commercial ecosystem has grown around these compounds. Some of it is people sharing what they believe helped them. Some of it is not.

Regulators publish guidance on this because the problem is longstanding, and the language used by fraudulent cancer products is remarkably consistent. The FDA lists specific phrases that should function as red flags, including claims that a product treats all forms of cancer, miraculously kills cancer cells and tumours, shrinks malignant tumours, selectively kills cancer cells while leaving healthy cells intact, is more effective than chemotherapy, or cures cancer [SRC-0043].

Read that list again with the material from this book in mind. Several of those phrases will be familiar.

The FDA also names the harm precisely, and it is not primarily the product.

Such products may appear harmless but can cause harm by delaying or interfering with proven, beneficial treatment [SRC-0043]. That is the same sequence Chapter 2 traced through the published case reports.

Beyond the vocabulary, some structural signals are worth knowing.

Selling and advising at the same time. A person who tells you what to take and also sells it to you has an interest in your conclusion. This does not make them wrong, and it does mean the advice needs checking elsewhere.

Payment for access rather than for care. Fees to join a group, to receive a protocol, or to access "investigational" treatment outside a trial.

Discouraging you from telling your oncologist. This is the clearest signal in this entire book. Anyone advising secrecy from your medical team is advising something that, on the evidence in Chapter 2, gets people hurt. There is no legitimate version of this advice.

Testimonials in place of data. Discussed at length in Chapters 2 and 3. A large number of accounts is not a small number of studies.

Urgency. Limited availability, prices rising, act now. Cancer decisions are rarely improved by speed, and legitimate medicine does not run on countdown timers.

Certainty that outruns the evidence. Anyone who is more confident about these compounds than the evidence in Chapters 2 and 3 supports is telling you something about themselves rather than about the compounds.

Discrediting the alternative rather than supporting the claim. Long passages about what is wrong with oncology, with little about what is right with the product. Chapter 2 examined the suppression argument and found a real observation inside it, but an argument about the system is not evidence about a compound.

None of this means that everyone discussing these compounds is dishonest. Most people sharing their experience are sincere. It means that between you and the evidence there is now an industry, and knowing its habits is part of reading anything it produces.

It is worth describing the opposite as well, because a list of warning signs can leave you unable to trust anything.

A source worth reading tends to do several things. It states what kind of evidence it is describing, and where the evidence came from, in enough detail that you could find it. It distinguishes between what has been shown in cells, in animals, and in people. It says what remains unknown, without treating uncertainty as a reason for either confidence or dismissal. It reports unfavourable findings alongside favourable ones. It has no financial interest in your conclusion, or it declares one. It tells you when it was last updated. And it is comfortable with you checking.

Government health agencies, major cancer organisations, and professional oncology societies generally meet that description, and their patient-facing material is written to be read by people in exactly your position. It is less exciting than what the algorithm serves you. It is also the material that is still accurate in a year.

A final word for anyone who has already spent money on this.

People do, sometimes a great deal, and the discovery that a source was not what it appeared to be lands hard on top of everything else. If that is you, two things are worth separating.

The money is gone or it is not, and that is a consumer question. Regulators in most countries take reports of fraudulent health claims, and reporting is worth doing even when recovery is unlikely, because enforcement actions are built from reports.

The medical question is entirely separate and more urgent. If you took something, the relevant step is telling your team, for all the reasons this book has set out. Embarrassment is a common reason people do not, and it is the worst possible reason, because the cost of silence falls on your treatment rather than on your pride.

WHERE THIS LEAVES YOU

You have a claim brief, a medication list, a set of anchored questions, and a map of who can answer what. That is a considerable amount more than most people bring.

It is worth being clear about what this preparation can and cannot achieve. It will not make an unproven compound proven. It will not guarantee a satisfying conversation, and it cannot make anyone give you certainty that does not exist.

What it does is ensure that the decision, whatever it turns out to be, is made with the fullest picture available to you, by the person entitled to make it, with the people who can see your actual situation informed and able to help.

That is the most that anyone in this position can arrange. It is also, genuinely, quite a lot.

It is worth noticing how much of this is transferable. The claim brief works on any health claim, not just these three compounds. The anchored questions work in any specialty. The medication picture is useful at every appointment you will ever attend. And knowing which member of a team answers which kind of question is a skill that outlasts any particular illness.

That is not a consolation prize. The claim that brought you here will eventually be replaced by another one, and the people around you will face versions of the same problem. What you have built in this chapter is the part that keeps working.

WHERE THIS LEADS

The work is done. What remains is shorter, and it concerns something this book has circled without naming directly.

Every reader who got this far did so because of hope, and hope has been treated throughout as something to be handled carefully. That is not the same as something to be discouraged.

The conclusion is about what hope looks like when it is attached to accurate information, and about the questions worth carrying forward when the next claim arrives. Because it will.

CHAPTER 6
WHAT TO CARRY WITH YOU

BACK TO THE LINK

This book began with someone sending you a link.

You have now spent a considerable amount of time on it. You have read about cells and mice and trials, about a laboratory accident in 2008, about a man in Oklahoma, about a retracted paper and a journal notice, about liver enzymes and a pump in the wall of a blood vessel. It has been a lot to hold.

So it is worth returning to that first moment and asking what has actually changed.

The claim in the link is still there. It has not been proved and it has not been disproved. If you went back and watched the video again tonight, it would make the same assertions in the same confident tone, and the comments underneath would still be full of people saying it saved their lives.

What has changed is you.

You can now read that video and see its structure. You can see where the story ends and the claim begins. You can see which rung of the ladder its evidence sits on, and how many rungs above that the claim has been placed. You can see whether the cited paper is about the compound being discussed. You can check, in about a minute, whether that paper still stands.

That is not a small thing. It is a different relationship to the whole subject, and it does not expire.

If you have been reading this on someone else's behalf, something else has changed too.

The introduction described you: the husband, the daughter, the friend who took on the job of reading everything so that someone else would not have to. That job was real work and you have now done a great deal of it.

What you can offer at the end of it is not a conclusion. It is something better and considerably harder to come by. You can hand over a page instead of a worry. You can say what is known and what is not, in a form the person can use. You can sit in the appointment and write down what was said. And you can do all of that without taking the decision away from the person it belongs to.

That was always the useful role. It is worth knowing that you have finished the part that was yours.

WHAT THE EVIDENCE CAME TO

It is worth stating the position once more, plainly, because it is easy to lose in the detail.

None of the three compounds has been shown to treat cancer in people. That is the finding, and every part of it earned its place.

Fenbendazole has laboratory activity in some models and not others, no characterised behaviour in the human body, no completed cancer trial, a retracted case series, and a growing set of published reports of liver injury.

Ivermectin has broad laboratory activity, a genuine and unresolved dispute among researchers about whether the concentrations involved are reachable in a person, and one small early-phase trial in which most evaluable patients progressed. A larger trial is planned. The question is open in the specific sense that someone is now asking it properly.

Mebendazole has the strongest preclinical case of the three and the most human evidence. When it was tested in a randomised trial against a benchmark set in advance, it did not meet it.

That last sentence is the one to sit with. The compound with the most evidence produced the clearest answer, and the answer was not the hoped-for one. Whatever else this subject is, it is not a case of nobody looking.

None of that means these compounds are worthless, or that the researchers studying them are wasting their time, or that you were foolish to ask. It means what it says, and no more.

It is also worth remembering that each of those verdicts was written so that it could change, and what would change it was set down at the time. A randomised trial meeting a predefined endpoint. Human pharmacokinetic data showing that meaningful concentrations are achievable. A study designed well enough that its result could be relied upon.

None of those things is impossible, and if any of them arrives, the position in this book becomes out of date. That is not a weakness in the argument. It is the difference between a conclusion and a conviction, and it is the standard the book has been asking you to apply to everything else.

WHAT HOPE IS FOR

There is a way of reading everything above as an instruction to stop hoping. That reading would be wrong, and it is worth spending the last pages on why.

Hope is not a belief that a particular compound will work. It never was. That is a claim, and claims can be checked, which is what this book has been doing.

Hope is something else, and it is more durable than any specific claim, which is fortunate, because specific claims fail all the time. Hope survives a negative trial. A conviction about a compound does not.

Consider what hope attached to accurate information can actually do. It can get you to the appointment with a page of questions rather than a vague dread. It can get you into a trial you would not have known about. It can get you to a palliative care team that makes the next six months substantially better than they would have been. It can keep you on a treatment that is working, rather than off it because something undisclosed damaged your liver and nobody could tell why.

Every one of those is a real outcome, available to you, and none requires anything to be proved first.

Now consider the alternative. Hope attached to a specific unproven claim has a particular shape. It burns brightly, it demands defending, and it breaks when the evidence arrives. And while it lasts it costs things: money, sometimes; attention, always; and occasionally the treatment that was actually working.

There is a version of this that is worth protecting rather than dismantling. Wanting there to be something. Being unwilling to accept that the current answer is the final one. Reading, asking, refusing to be passive. That impulse is why some of the research described in this book exists at all, and it is not the enemy of accuracy. It is what accuracy is for.

The distinction is simply this. Hope is a way of facing forward. It is not a method for deciding what is true.

WHAT THIS BOOK DID NOT DO

It did not tell you what to take. That was not caution; it was the honest limit of what any book can know about a particular person.

It did not tell you that everyone in white coats is right, or that everyone questioning them is wrong. Chapter 2 examined the argument that cheap drugs go unstudied and found something true inside it. Chapter 3 found a randomised trial that was run, published, and negative. Both of those are what the evidence looks like, and neither fits a simple story about who to trust.

And it did not promise you certainty. There is not much of it available here, and a book that manufactured some would have been easier to read and worse for you.

What it gave you instead was a way of working. That may feel like less than you wanted when you started. It is more than you will get from the next video, and unlike the video, it will still be true next year.

The Five Questions

Everything in this book reduces to five questions. They are the Claim Check from the introduction, in the form you will actually use them. They work on any health claim, from any source, about anything.

One. What exactly is being claimed?

Write it as a single sentence, with the story removed. If you cannot, the claim may be too vague to check, and that is your answer.

Two. Which compound, and in what situation?

Which one, specifically. Human medicine or veterinary product. Alone or alongside treatment. For days or for months. In which cancer, at which stage. Missing details are not gaps in your knowledge. They are usually gaps in the claim.

Three. What kind of evidence is this, and what did it actually measure?

Cells, animals, one person, a group, or a trial. Then separately: tumours shrunk, symptoms improved, or people living longer. The distance between the claim and the measurement is usually the whole story.

Four. What else could explain it, and has anything changed since?

Was there a comparison group. Was something else happening at the same time. And has the paper been corrected, questioned, or withdrawn since it was published.

Five. What is the one question I should bring to my team?

This is the step that turns reading into something useful. Everything before it is preparation for this.

Five questions. A few minutes. They will not tell you what to do, and they were never designed to. What they do is replace a feeling with an account, and an account is something you can act on.

THE LAST THING

The next claim is already being filmed.

It may be about a different compound. The video will be well made, the reference list will look solid, and someone who cares about you will send it. That is not a cynical prediction. It is simply what happens when large numbers of frightened people are looking for something and other people have noticed.

When it arrives, you will know what to do with it. Not dismiss it, and not swallow it. Take it apart, find out what is actually known, and bring the remainder to someone who can see your situation.

One final word, and it is the most important thing here.

Whatever you decide, the decision belongs to you. Not to a video, not to a family member who is frightened, not to a stranger selling something, and not to this book. You are entitled to weigh uncertainty differently than someone else would. You are entitled to disagree with your oncologist. You are entitled to change your mind.

What this book has tried to give you is not an answer. It is the ability to make that decision with your eyes open, knowing what is known, what is not, and who to ask about the difference.

That is what was available, and it is what an honest book on this subject could offer. I hope it is useful.

One last practical note. If someone you know receives a diagnosis, this material will be relevant to them within about a week, and they will be reading at two in the morning like everyone else. The five questions travel. So does the claim brief, and so does the habit of saving a link before it disappears. None of it requires them to read this book first.

The appendices that follow contain the tools in portable form: a glossary, the evidence key, the claim brief, the medication list, the question sets, a trial checklist, a way to check a paper's status, and a page for whoever is helping you. They are meant to be printed, written on, and taken to appointments.

www.ingramcontent.com/pod-product-compliance
Lightning Source LLC
LaVergne TN
LVHW060042210926
848481LV00013B/3937
* 9 7 8 1 9 5 6 5 7 0 9 2 2 *